Naturopathy

Evolve to the Alternate Form of
Naturopathic Medicine

*(Everything You Need to Know About
Naturopathic Medicine)*

Leroy Somers

Published By **Bengion Cosalas**

Leroy Somers

All Rights Reserved

Naturopathy: Evolve to the Alternate Form of Naturopathic Medicine (Everything You Need to Know About Naturopathic Medicine)

ISBN 978-1-77485-747-2

No part of this guidebook shall be reproduced in any form without permission in writing from the publisher except in the case of brief quotations embodied in critical articles or reviews.

Legal & Disclaimer

The information contained in this ebook is not designed to replace or take the place of any form of medicine or professional medical advice. The information in this ebook has been provided for educational & entertainment purposes only.

The information contained in this book has been compiled from sources deemed reliable, and it is accurate to the best of the Author's knowledge; however, the Author cannot guarantee its accuracy and validity and cannot be held liable for any errors or omissions. Changes are periodically made to this book. You must consult your doctor or get professional medical advice before using any of the suggested remedies, techniques, or information in this book.

Upon using the information contained in this book, you agree to hold harmless the Author from and against any damages, costs, and expenses, including any legal fees potentially resulting from the application of any of the information provided by this guide. This disclaimer applies to any damages or injury caused by the use and application, whether directly or indirectly, of any advice or information presented, whether for breach of contract, tort, negligence, personal injury, criminal intent, or under any other cause of action.

You agree to accept all risks of using the information presented inside this book. You need to consult a professional medical practitioner in order to ensure you are both able and healthy enough to participate in this program.

Table Of Contents

Chapter 1: The Types Of Naturopathic Treatments _____1

Chapter 2: Reiki Energy Healing____17

Chapter 3: Manipulation (Chiropractic, Osteopathic, Etc)____45

Chapter 4: The Benefits Of Naturopathy _____62

Chapter 5: Faq About Naturopathy 73

Chapter 6: The Philosophy Behind Naturopathy _____76

Chapter 7: Homeopathy_____105

Chapter 8: Self-Study Assessment 146

Conclusion _____183

Chapter 1: The Types Of Naturopathic Treatments

"Naturopathy" is a term used to describe a variety of treatments "Naturopathy" can be used to refer to a range of treatments. Actually, some of the most sought-after holistic health treatments like massage and chiropractic, are both Naturopathic therapies. Here are a few of the Naturopathy methods you might think about when starting your holistic plan of treatment:

Ayurveda

Ayurveda has been practiced for hundreds of years. It first became popular in India in the region of India, where it was used to aid in restoring the body's equilibrium and to treat various illnesses. Ayurvedic practitioners are based on the notion that wellness can only be maintained when there is equilibrium between our body mind , and spirit. Ayurvedic Medicine can be an essential element of your preventative treatment, and can be used to treat specific medical conditions when used in conjunction with a whole-body treatment regimen.

If you see an Avurvedic practitioner for the first time, he'll conduct an evaluation of your overall health. He will seek out areas that may be in need of attention instead of providing an assessment based on the specific symptoms you experience. For instance, in your initial appointment the doctor will examine your speech patterns and condition of your tongue and also inquire about a range of questions regarding your eating habits and lifestyle.

Ayurveda is based on the notion of, as many Naturopathic treatments do that we're all composed of five elements. They combine to form the three vital life energy sources that are pitta dosha, vata dosha, and kapha. It is believed that these three energetic forces are responsible for all aspects of our body and determine the way it operates. The method suggested by your doctor will depend on which energy is causing the imbalance.

The Avurvedic practitioner could choose to utilize a range of treatments and techniques, like massage and specially blended teas used to cleanse the body, oils, as well as blood. The practitioner will usually offer suggestions on how you can improve your health at your own pace by incorporating meditation as part of your day-to-day routine or using aromatherapy to boost your energy every morning, for instance.

It is evident that the vast majority of Ayurvedic practitioners adhere to certain guidelines, all of which aid in improving the health and wellbeing of patients. Since Ayurveda is a practice that involves energy sources located within our bodies, these guidelines are designed to assist in balance between the three kinds of energy. Here are a few "rules" that a lot of Naturopaths and Ayurvedic practitioners should bear in their minds:

Beware of any junk food including processed foods and foods that have an excessive amount of additives, fats or sugars.

Avoid eating regularly. In general the Ayurvedic practitioner will break up three meals and at least a 3 hour gap between them.

It is recommended that you avoid staying awake late at late at night. This will enable the body the right amount of sleep it requires to maintain an energy level that is optimal.

- Exercise is essential. However, it is not recommended to exercise after eating an meal.

If you are hungry between meals, be able to satisfy that craving by eating fruit or juices that are fresh (not junk food or fried foods).

It is essential to ensure that you don't miss meals, and also be careful not to overeat.

People who receive Ayurvedic medicines are usually advised to stay clear of animal products (animal protein). In lieu, eating a balanced diet consisting of vegetables, sprouts, herbs and pulses are recommended.

Do not eat meals that are either too hot or cold. Additionally, don't put your body in extreme temperature.

Do regular (or every week) massage with oils that contain herbs. As well as a complete body massage, you must be massaging on your scalp with the oil since it can improve circulation.

You can participate in regular meditation, yoga or any other relaxing exercises.

In addition to the Ayurvedic guidelines here are a few ideas I'd like give you on how you can make maximum benefit from your Ayurvedic life style:

Get up early so that you can be able to enjoy your day to the maximum. If you're able to fall asleep at the time you need to (no after 10pm) and you're able to sleep in, then you might be able to rise at 5 or 4 am. If you do get up in the morning, take a moment to breathe deeply and think about the day ahead prior to kicking off your day.

Consume as many seasonal fresh vegetables and fruits as you can throughout your meals. This will enable your body to cleanse and detoxify, particularly if you steer clear of all oily, high-fat foods (such like fast foods).

Try taking an ounce of water each 30 minutes or so and ensure the water temperature is not too high. This will help ensure that your body is well-hydrated.

You must engage in regular exercises However, don't do it too much. After you're done exercising in a strenuous routine exercises, it's a good option to engage in some type of relaxation routine.

When you are preparing your weekly menu Focus on simple meals. Additionally, while eating, make sure to be as relaxed as you can. make sure that you create a peaceful environment surrounding you. That means you shouldn't be watching TV when eating.

Eat only whenever you're actually hungry. We tend to snack because it's the time that we're used too, or during social gatherings, or simply due to boredom. According to Ayurveda generally it is best to eat at times when hungry. However it is important to not skipping breakfast as is the most significant food of the day.

Do not eat anything heavy before going to go to bed. If you feel feeling hungry, consider eating vegetables or fruits or drink juices.

According to Ayurveda It's a good practice to detoxify as the seasons change. Therefore, when the new season is on the horizon, it's recommended to eat light foods as well as drink lots of water that is room temperature (or slightly warmer). It can also help aid in digestion.

Try to take bathing as often as feasible, with warm water. Additionally, add the drops of your preferred essential oil to help relax and rejuvenate your mind and body.

Yoga

Although Yoga is not the practitioner performing procedures, it's thought to be a type that is a form of Naturopathic healing. It is based on the body's ability of healing itself and helps improve your body's systems and boost your energy levels by performing a series of specific actions. There are many various types of yoga you can pick from and each one has each of their own advantages. But, all kinds of Yoga are designed with the same purpose in mind which is to find balance between your body and mind and also to increase you mental clarity as well as increase your overall health.

Yoga can reduce stress levels as well as improve your ability to perceive. It may even aid in becoming more aware of your body , and improve your overall well-being. Yoga has been practiced in India for centuries, however, it's now becoming increasingly well-known all over the world. In actual fact, it's considered to be one of the most effective ways that offer holistic health.

To find the kind of Yoga that is right for you it's best to explore a variety of the different types of Yoga. Each type has its own benefits and benefits, and you might need to employ a range of different methods in you Yoga routine. This is a brief outline of a few Yoga methods you might be interested in:

Vinyasa. This form of yoga is focused on synchronizing your breathing and your movements. Vinyasa includes a sequence of 12 postures that are often referred to as the "sun salutation" where all your movements are linked to the rhythm of your breathing. It aids in increasing your muscle mass, boosts the strength of your muscles, and improves flexibility. It can also lower your chance of developing various diseases or health issues, including heart disease, hypertension, and health issues related to stress.

Hatha. This type of yoga was developed in the 15th century. It is ideal for those who are new to yoga because of its focus on the most basic postures as well as relaxation methods, specifically in comparison to other types of yoga. It helps to decrease stress, improve your physical well-being and improve your breathing and improve your life quality.

Bikram. This type of yoga is thought to be one of the most challenging types of yoga due to the fact that it is practiced in rooms with temperatures ranging from 95 to 100 degrees Fahrenheit. It is the reason why it has been dubbed "hot yoga." It consists of 26 postures that are all designed to strengthen muscles and eliminate the toxins located within your body. It's great for those who want to lose some weight and recover from injuries or cleanse their general system.

Ashtanga. This kind of yoga is sometimes known as "power yoga" because of its fact that it is an intense physical effort and more complex exercises like push ups and lunges. It is practiced at a more fast speed. It can help reduce stress, boosts your mental health and can even help with your efforts to lose weight.

Iyengar. This kind of yoga usually uses various pieces of equipment , or "props" that include straps or blocks to help you align your body and build strength. Contrary to other kinds of yoga, most of the Iyengar's exercises require you stay in a standing posture. It aids in improving the balance of your body and is ideal for those recovering from surgery or injury.

There are many things that could interfere with practicing Yoga throughout the day. Believe me when I say (from my own experiences) that you might find yourself exhausted after working for a long time or doing chores around the home and unable to squeeze Yoga in your daily schedule. Maybe you believe you're not physically fit enough to master the techniques that Yoga demands. But I can tell you that anyone can get any benefit from practicing yoga whatever age you are, health or weight. Even if you live an extremely busy lifestyle it is important to find just a few minutes to engage in some yoga. It's only some time from your schedule, and is worth the effort and time you spend.

Meditation

Meditation can provide your body with the chance to unwind and recharge its self. It also permits you to have the time your mind and body need to heal and to improve your overall health. There's no particular method of meditation, nor how to go about it. There are a myriad of kinds of meditation including some that simply require just sitting in silence for only a few minutes a day, while others suggest that you change your way of life. The type you pick is based on your individual preferences, and the amount of time you'd like to commit to your meditation.

If you are just beginning your meditation practice you should try to set aside at least a few minutes every day to pay attention to your thoughts and focus on your breathing in a mindful way. Meditation practitioners believe that it is important to make time for yourself to allow your mind and body to reconnect and heal. It also lets you contemplate your feelings and the events of your day. It is suggested that when you are trying to meditate you take a seat in a peaceful location free of distractions. Although some forms of meditation require to concentrate on your thoughts and alter your breathing pattern and others might require you repeat a mantra or positive affirmation.

There are many kinds of meditationavailable, it's beneficial to test a variety of techniques to discover the one that is most effective for you. This gives you the chance to truly experience the various methods employed for each, before choosing the one you consider to be the most beneficial. Here are a few examples of the many different types of meditation you could think about:

Transcendental. The type of meditation that transcends tends to be more complex than the other forms you'll see in this list. If you are practicing transcendental meditation, it is common to sit with your back in a perfect alignment and practice the mantra (a particular word or phrase that you've written for yourself) in the course of meditation. The principal purpose for transcendental meditation is to release anything that is only temporary as well as be able to "rise" above all else. Most often, practitioners seek to attain a different state of consciousness, that is, they might quit their physical body. This kind of meditation isn't primarily focused on helping you find your purpose in life, or to overcome any emotional difficulties you might have however, it is a way to connect with your "universal power" that is beyond the mind and body.

Guided Imagery. During a guided image meditation (also called guide visualization, or guided meditation) session, you're guided to visualize a tranquil landscape that will help you relax and achieve inner peace. If, for instance, you're stressed due to your work You could think of sitting on a serene beach, bathed in sunshine, listening to the waves and imagine the scenery for a couple of minutes. To effectively practice this kind of meditation, seek out a peaceful space in your home or outside, particularly one that is devoid of distractions that could make it difficult to fully the most benefit from your imagined location. If you find it difficult to attain peaceful state of mind when you participate in the guided imagery practice There are plenty of audio recordings available online that you can enjoy which can assist you in learning to visualize a specific scene. These recordings will allow you to visualize a peaceful and tranquil environment, even in the event that your life is somewhat stress-inducing in the present.

Zazen. This kind of therapy requires that you lie in one place for a prolonged duration. It's a minimalist kind of holistic therapy to put it lightly. There isn't much direction provided on how the practice should be conducted however it is generally thought that you should concentrate in your position and repeat a certain mantra or phrase throughout your session. Zazen could be difficult for people who are just beginning, because there's no method that should be performed. This could be a challenge for those who prefer the structure or instruction in their practice of meditation. Also, unlike many kinds practices, Zazen isn't focused on the breathing patterns you use. In fact, the practitioners aren't required to alter their breathing at all throughout their sessions.

Kundalini. The concept of this type of meditation is that there is a flow of energy that flows through us, as being a multitude of energy centers that are located in our bodies. In Kudalini meditations, you're instructed to concentrate on the rising stream of energy, and then move it towards your body heat by breathing each breath. The main goal is to let the stream to as high as it could, and to attempt to raise the energy towards a point which is right below your hairline (which is also known as the center of energy).

Qi Gong. While Kundalini relies on breath to push energy upwards, Qi Gong utilizes breath to shift energies through your body in an oval motion. In Qi Gong, there are three energy points that are specific to you, each of which is focussed on during the meditation practice.

Be aware that these are only some of the various types of meditation. If you don't find one that is appealing to you There's an abundance of information available in holistic healing books as well as on the internet on the various types of meditation and the benefits they bring.

As I've been practicing meditation for years I thought it would be beneficial to share a few of techniques I've learned throughout my journey:

Choose comfortable clothing for meditation. I strongly suggest wearing loose-fitting clothes or an outfit you are comfortable in when practicing your meditations. In actuality, it could be prudent to invest in an outfit only designated for "meditation clothes".

Try to stay in the present and enjoy every day. While you're in meditation do not think about what you're going to do when you've completed your meditation, or what you're not going to be able to accomplish when you've added this practice to your already hectic schedule. If you're in a state of meditation it is important to just be in the present and try not to let other thoughts take over your thoughts. This will help you get the most out of every day by taking moment to unwind from the stresses and thoughts you've collected.

Make sure you set aside time to meditate each day. You should set aside a time every day when you can do your meditation, no matter what it might mean. For instance, if find that you have extra time to meditate in the morning before the rest of the world wakes up, then you can set the time for your meditation and record it on your calendar.

has even been used to heal rituals and as a means of expression since as long as the beginning of time. In all time art has been used to heal ailments and offer emotional relief. There are some traditions who make and wear masks which are believed to have the power of animals and to deter evil forces. The growing awareness of naturopathy and alternative therapies has led to its increasing popularity in recent times. Nowadays, art therapy helps us achieve an enlightened state of mind and can even change our way of feeling and think.

To provide you with an idea of what you could be able to experience during a typical therapy appointment, below are some options of instruments that may be employed during an appointment with an experienced therapist:

Masks. They are among the oldest tools of art currently available. If you let people create or wear masks of their choice you give them the freedom to express themselves freely without being marginalized or criticized, due to the fact that they can temporarily to transform into a different persona. In therapy sessions with art in general, the client will be asked to create the mask (or select one from a selection) which best represents his personal circumstances or emotions. The patient will then be able to display the true feelings and thoughts.

Mandalas. Mandalas, the Sanskrit term used to describe "sacred circles" and have been used throughout time to aid in meditation. Tibetan Monks have created Mandalas from sand for a long time and the process of creating Mandalas is believed to be a type of meditation in itself. These symbols aid us in focusing our attention and concentrate on the most important things in our lives and assist in focusing our energies. If you allow your patients to design their own Mandala in an art therapy session that is transpersonal it allows them to be more open and understand their needs and also put them in touch to their own inner self. Therapists even advise their clients to keep Mandala journals in which they can write down their feelings and reflect on their life experiences.

Dreams. In reality, dreams can also be utilized as a tool for the transpersonal art therapy sessions. If you truly consider the nature of dreams and what they represent, they could be interpreted as a flow of visual images that flow direct from our unconscious which reflect our actual emotions and thoughts. In the course of an art therapy the therapist could have the patient draw the outline of a current or frequent dream she is experiencing, and then to discuss what the dream could mean. This could help the patient be more precise in interpreting her dreams in terms of what they are and determine the reason they are happening to her and also how they could aid her in changing her life.

Clay. Clay is a product of the earth, and therefore can be an excellent tool to use for therapy who need energetic and grounding. It will help you get more at peace, and offer you the opportunity to express any feelings that you might be experiencing. This is particularly true for patients who are tactile, meaning people prefer speaking through their hands. Clay can also help you create a 3-D picture, that can better communicate your thoughts and emotions.

Paint as well as Canvas (or other art media). Therapists may choose to allow his patients to work on the canvas using oil paints or watercolours. In most cases, this permits the patients to be expressive with no any limitations, as they have a blank canvas and can release any hidden emotions or worries they might be feeling.

The most important aspect you must remember about the art of therapy is each patient is unique. What is effective for you might not be the same for another. So, finding the therapist you're at ease with and who provides an approach you believe is most effective is essential.

Sound Therapy

Sound therapy professionals will employ various auditory stimuli to assist their patients deal with emotional issues that could be affecting their physical well-being. Gongs and singing bowls from the past are used in the session, as in the form of musical recordings. The primary objective of the use of sound therapy is to bring peace and self-healing. It is also a way to help with a variety of health problems like ADHD and ongoing back discomfort, headaches and migraines. You could perform sound therapy at home, in which you lie in a peaceful space that is free of distractions, and then listen to gentle music (classical is advised).

There's a kind which has been becoming increasingly popular in recent times that is called "binaural beats" (or in other words, binaural sounds). They were first discovered in 1839, however they are only beginning to be popular in the past few years. They are believed to be a part of the process that are able to help you reach an increased state of relaxation and they are believed to have the ability to increase creativity. They are also used as a tool for meditation.

In essence, binaural beats can be best described as a type of sound. For instance, if you were to play a sound into your ear that was 250 Hz, and another in the opposite ear was 270 Hz then it would create a binaural rhythm of 20 Hz. If this happens your brain will interpret it as a pulsing tone like that the sounds playing in both ears were mixed. It is considered that binaural beats provide a range of effects in addition including the capacity to decrease anxiety and aid people to focus.

If you're looking to give the binaural beats a go There are plenty of recordings to discover on the internet. Find a quiet area in your home (free from distractions) and use earphones for maximum results. It is possible that you can attain a state of relaxation , and may even rest better at night.

Consultations on Nutrition

A consultation with a Nutritional Therapist can be a fantastic method to integrate Naturopathy into your health program. Every food item we consume is broken into pieces by our bodies in order to supply us with energy. The fact is that everything that we consume is absorbed into our cells, and directly affects our physical and mental health. In the end food has the capacity to boost or degrade your health. A visit to a nutritionist will allow you to alter your diet and get an understanding of what foods are best for you.

In a typical appointment during a typical consultation, the Nutritionist will review the current habits you are eating and advise you on which foods are suitable to add to your food regimen. This will allow you to enhance your health, aid you lose weight and may even improve how you feel. A lot of Naturopathic doctors include Nutritional consultations as part of their treatment plans.

Even people who aren't obese and have a relatively healthy lifestyle could benefit from a nutritional consultation. For instance, people who've lived a healthy life and are now experiencing medical issues can go to a professional who will assist them in adjusting their diets. The consultant will provide alternatives to your food choices If you're looking for ways to be healthier (and not become bored of the standard "diet" food choices) and also provide you with new recipes. A lot of people schedule an appointment with a nutritionist every year (typically after annual health checks) in order to be able to tweak their diet in order to address any health issues identified during the examination.

Here are a few conditions which can be treated or treated with the help of an experienced nutritionist:

Heart disease or health concerns

The cause is high blood pressure (hypertension)

- The levels of cholesterol are high.

Celiac disease

Certain food-related allergies

Irritable bowel syndrome (also called IBS)

Pre-diabetic and diabetes health issues

Weight gain - sudden or extreme weight increase

Infertility or pregnancy issues

When you first meet with a nutritionist you'll typically discuss your goals as well as the main motives behind seeking advice on your diet. The consultant might also ask you to provide your medical history along with any medications you might be taking. You will then talk about your way of life, which could include not just what you're eating, but also the amount of stress you're feeling as well as how much sleep you get as well as how energetic you are.

It is common for people to be asked to keep a food journal where you note all your meals between meetings. You may also keep an eye on your exercise routine in your diary. Some experts will suggest you to write down your feelings as well to help you get an understanding of your current emotional state.

Unani

Unani is an Naturopathic treatment method that was developed in Greece in Greece, and is referred to as Unan. Unani is among only a few holistic treatment techniques that do not involve medication, which aid the body's self-healing process. Based on the principles of Unani the ailments we experience are part of the bodies "natural process" and the symptoms that we feel are the result of how our bodies handle the natural processes. The body is able to maintain itself, which assists us maintain our equilibrium. In essence, Unani is designed to assist our bodies to restore the equilibrium that naturally happens by identifying and addressing the four main indicators of imbalance. These comprise of balgham (phlegm) and Safra (yellow bile) as well as dum (blood) as well as sauda (black bile).

If you seek the assistance of an Unani practitioner Your pulse will be checked along with the stool and urine in certain cases. The treatment plan you receive will be based on results. Drugs that are potent aren't recommended in the beginning, and lower doses of medications are typically utilized throughout.

Color Therapy

In spite of the fact that a lot of us are familiar with the colors we see around us, the colours play a significant part in the overall well-being of our bodies and minds. They help us heal physically and emotionally as well as improve the overall health of our bodies and minds. Colors have the ability to make you feel positive, much like painting your room at home with a new color could cause you to feel more comfortable. If you pay attention to the colors that you pick, you'll can directly affect your well-being.

Therapists are trained in the practice of Chromotherapy. In a chromotherapy session patients are exposed that are of various colors in order to improve their overall well-being. Chromotherapy, also known as colour therapy, is based on notion that colours are able to affect our energy and emotions. Because we are visual creatures humans are able to associate certain colours with moods or emotions. For instance, when a lot of us see blue light it brings thoughts of peace and tranquility. However, orange could bring us a sense of vitality. So, if we're looking to boost our feelings of tranquility, an orange bedroom can trigger an unwelcome reaction and hinder our ability to sleep soundly.

The use of colour therapy will allow you to understand which colors can offer the greatest benefit and allow for you to integrate these colors in your daily routine. So, seeking the assistance of a color therapist will help you get the most benefit from this holistic approach to healing.

To make you aware of the impact that certain colours can have an array of emotions (and are able to be used in your daily life to provide you with the ability to change your outlook) I'll present an explanation of every one of the popular colours that you'll see every day. This is a brief review of what the most well-known colors represent and how they can be used to create particular moods or feelings:

Blue: Increases feelings of peace and calm. This is also the color which symbolizes honesty, truth and sincerity. It may be beneficial to choose blue if facing a stressful situation or are trying to get calm with those who can cause frustration or tension.

Violetsymbolizes the ability to think and feel. It's also the perfect color to incorporate into designs of the meditation space because it is the symbol of the universal flow of energy.

Red can be a great boost in energy levels. It can also boost energy and vitality and enthusiasm. This is the color is the one to choose when you're in search of an exciting new color in your bedrooms (especially in the event that you feel your relationship needs an extra spark).

OrangeThe color orange Boosts your creativity and increases your optimism. It's popular for its capacity to increase emotion, productivity and enjoyment. The best choice is orange if experiencing a negative mood or are suffering from the symptoms of a creative problem (such the writer's block).

Green- It is the color of harmony and balance. It also represents love, nature and the ability to communicate with family and friends. Green is an excellent color to consider when you live in a chaotic and chaotic or if you're having issues with people who are around you frequently.

YellowIt is the colour of humour and fun. It also represents intellect self-confidence, personal strength and logical thinking. If you're struggling with depression or boredom You can easily fix your situation by incorporating a splash of sunshine into your daily life.

I'd like to also share some of the ways I incorporate color therapy into my everyday routine. You can totally change your perspective on life simply by adding a touch of colour in a few places. There are numerous ways to do this, aside from going to color therapy sessions. Here are some ways I have used colour to make my life better:

If you're going to take an bath, why don't you add a few colored bath salts in the hot water?

This will help reduce tension and ease tight muscles (especially when you are using Epsom salts) as well as boost your mood. I highly suggest you try one of these color therapy baths after having an especially tough day, or prior to any event that is stressful.

If you're like a lot of people, you're likely to spend a significant amount of your time at home. Even if you're absent more frequently than you'd prefer, you likely still view it as a place where you can unwind from the this world, for just a time. Why do you want to paint the walls of your house to create various moods? If, for instance, you're seeking an option for your room to be more peaceful and relaxing, paint your walls blue.

Wear clothes with appropriate for the color you wish to change how you feel throughout your day. It can be a beneficial influence on those around you which can be a major benefit. If, for instance, you know you're likely to be dealing with someone who's not a good friend this day, don the yellow tie or scarf since this color is a symbol of fun and laughter.

Buy lamps with colored shades and set them in your home. This allows the room to take on this particular color without having paint the walls. This is an excellent alternative if you don't wish to change the color of your space, and only want to create the effect of colour therapy quickly. It's not even mentioning that this is a cheaper option to alter the colour the walls.

Create drinks that have been colored. There are numerous flavored water additives can be purchased that come with several bright colors. If you're experiencing fatigue at work Why not bring red-colored water into your office to boost the energy level?

Buy food items that have of a specific colour and prepare your meal around these. For instance, if you want to prepare for an event you're not looking at, you might think about eating an orange prior to going out because this color can make you feel more positive.

If everything else fails and you're still not in a position to accurately represent the color, simply imagine the colour that best matches your mood. This is possible anywhere even in a crowded workplace or when you walk down the street. It can instantly make a big change in your attitude and perception.

Chinese Herbal Medicine

Chinese Herbal Medicine relies upon the idea that we should maintain the harmony between our body, mind and soul in order to keep our well-being. In lieu of fixing a particular illness the practitioners usually try to stop the illness from ever arising, by making sure that you're constantly maintaining a healthy equilibrium. Chinese Herbal Medicine uses a variety of herbs, and all provide a specific advantage or function. For instance even though one particular extract or herb could be beneficial for people who suffer from hypertension, another may be beneficial for those suffering from diabetes or abnormal blood sugar.

Since each herb has an impact and impact, it is highly recommended that you seek the assistance of a certified Chinese Herbal Medicine practitioner, instead of attempting to experiment with different herbs. There are more than 400 formulas used for Chinese Herbal Medicine, with some formulas containing as many twelve ingredients, or greater. This means that choosing the best combination of minerals and herbs is a exact science.

The traditional Chinese Medicine practitioner will carry through a thorough assessment prior to offering you the tea powder, tincture or pill that is most effectively for your needs. Prior to determining the right combination an assessment by your doctor usually includes a thorough review of your health and symptoms and an examination of your body. In this exam your eyes, ears the pulse, your skin hair and voice will be examined.

Reflexology

Reflexology is an Naturopathic healing technique that may help treat various medical conditions that include chronic pain. The practitioner applies gentle pressure to certain areas on the feet and hands of patients, as well as the ear, in some cases. There is a belief that these areas directly relate to an organ or system inside the body. If these points are stimulated in the area they are linked to benefit from a variety different health-related benefits. For instance If a specific area on the foot is believed to have a connection to digestion Patients may find that symptoms of Irritable Bowel are relieved.

In general, Reflexology isn't used to diagnose any issues and isn't believed as an "cure-all" for illnesses. However, it can be utilized as a part of an overall treatment program. Most often, patients employ other therapies in conjunction with Reflexology. For instance, massage or aromatherapy can be utilized as part of this holistic treatment for healing. An average Reflexology session begins with a thorough examination of your health history and an assessment of what issues or health issues Reflexology might be able assist you with.

A qualified practitioner will explain all the essentials of the Reflexology session prior to your appointment and will explain what happens during the session and what you might be expecting to experience. They'll also usually request that you sign a consent or health form, so make sure you arrive for the first appointment early in order to be able to complete this. Don't be afraid of asking questions regarding your treatment. You should feel like you are in a constant line of communication with your therapist.

After all the required documentation is completed and all concerns have been answered the doctor will generally request that you lie on the table for massage (or any other surface they normally utilize) and then begin work on a specific area of your body (feet hands, hands or ears). While certain ailments might react to treatment done with the feet, some will only react when pressure is applied to a specific area or hand. So, the therapist will focus on the area they feel is most appropriate to the issues you are facing. The health conditions you have may restrict the areas they concentrate on. For example, if you have a hand injury that has caused bruising or feet, they could focus with your feet instead.

Some reflexologists may also soak your feet before the treatment and rub your hands with specific oils. It's important to know that reflexologists typically conduct a brief examination of the health of your feet and hands at this point so that they can ensure the absence of visible wounds that might hinder the treatment. They'll also inquire whether you're experiencing any discomfort in these regions. Throughout the entire session, it is important to keep in contact with your therapist, letting them know of any areas that are aching or feel uneasy.

Throughout the treatment the therapist will employ various methods. They typically work on both feet and hands (and sometimes , the ears) as well as work on various points. A full session, which is designed to refine your body and strengthen your entire system, will involve work on every part of your feet and hands. This allows the hands and feet to be beneficial to all your internal organs muscles, nerves, muscle groups and bones. If they discover that a specific area is tight or painful it is common for them to apply pressure to the area to bring equilibrium to the region in the body. The primary objective of reflexology isn't to ease pain or tension which is felt at that important point, but rather to restore your body back to its normal equilibrium.

During the session, you might be experiencing a range of symptoms that will depend on the type of treatment you are receiving and your response to the treatment. Certain people are able to detect the area they are working with when they press the points. Others experience a feeling of lightness or dizziness.

Certain patients have noticed that they can feel energy moving through them after the obstruction is eliminated by the practitioner and notice that their mind and body are more in sync. Other reactions that can be experienced are:

The hand or foot area

The body temperature fluctuates

Congestion or coughing

Release of emotions (laughing or crying)

Changes in breath

Inability to remain alert (can't maintain your focus)

Thirst

After the therapist is finished working on the feet, hands or ears, they typically end the session with an energy-grounding method. This could involve gentle strokes or even a few minutes of quiet and focused breathing. It is important to feel at ease and secure during the entire treatment, regardless of when the treatment is nearing its end. It's usually an excellent idea to perform a short practice of grounding, like sitting for a short time or taking time to concentrate on the results that you've experienced during your Reflexology session by focusing on your body.

Do not rush off from the table. Take the time to unwind and recover after your session before getting up. If you notice any unusual symptoms it is important to bring it up to your doctor. There are a few adverse consequences (a significant majority are positive) that could occur from the reflexology treatment you received, for example:

- Increased energy and more restful sleep

- Pain relief

- Improved mobility

Tiredness or fatigue

- Skin eruptions (which result from the flushing of toxic substances)

Frequent stool movements (which is your body's method of eliminating toxic substances)

• Increased production of mucus

In general the average Reflexology session can last between 30-60 minutes, depending on the concerns you have and any issues you may have. After your treatment, you might want to take a few minutes to relax prior to leaving the office so that you can give you the chance to fully enjoy the results from the therapy. Drink plenty of water as Reflexology can assist in eliminating toxic substances, and being hydrated can allow the toxic substances to be easier to eliminated out of your body.

The reflexologist is likely to ask you to return for a subsequent session when a health issue is identified or to ensure that your body operating at peak levels. This is because the effects of Reflexology are usually subtle and the effects are gradually absorbed with time. It is therefore crucial to adhere to an appointment schedule and regularly visit your Therapist. If you're suffering from a specific illness that requires you to visit more often or even weekly for a certain number of weeks.

Acupuncture

Acupuncture has been utilized in the ancient times of China for hundreds of years. It is now being used as a holistic approach to healing and preventative treatment for medical conditions across the Western World too. Acupuncturists utilize small, sterilized needles that are inserted in specific areas of the body. As Reflexology points are linked to different organs and systems and organs, so do the points involved in the Acupuncture treatment.

There are two ways to approach Acupuncture one being The Western method of thinking as well as the traditional Eastern method. A lot of Western doctors believe needles are used to stimulate the nervous system and stimulate the tissues and muscles in order that patients may experience improved circulation and less discomfort. On the other hand traditional Chinese medical practitioners believe that acupuncture helps balance the flow of energy through the body. They believe that inserting needles into specific locations helps to bring balance back to the meridians of energy in your body.

Chapter 3: Manipulation (Chiropractic, Osteopathic, Etc)

There are many Manipulation treatments that are based on Naturopathic principles. Here are some of the most popular kinds of manipulative treatments you might want to take into consideration:

Chiropractic Treatment. Chiropractic care is based on the notion that your body is able to regulate and heal itself and adjusts your body in as to allow it to do this more effectively. It is believed that the spine, the brain as well as your nervous system comprise the primary components of the body that allow it to recover itself. Chiropractic treatments help to identify any issues with the spinal column as well as its structure, and assist to lessen the impact they can have on your nervous system as well as the general well-being of your body. This is done by moving the body's alignment, and fixing any problems that might be present in your skeletal system.

Physiotherapy. The Physiotherapist is of the belief that the body's movements play a vital part in the overall health of your. In an average Physiotherapy session, exercises manual therapy, physiotherapy, and electrophysical techniques can be employed by the therapist. The patient is fully engaged in their own health care and the therapist will assist the patient to improve their functioning and overall health.

Myopractics. Manipulation therapy assists patients in achieving better health and relieve chronic pain. In a typical session of Myopractic the practitioner will evaluate the patient's posture to identify areas where adjustments may require to be made. The goal of the treatment is to improve the structure of the body and return it to its natural form. Practitioners will attempt to determine where joints or bones might be in disarray, and then identify the muscle accountable for the disalignment. Once the muscle is removed then the joint or skeletal problem will be solved.

Hydrotherapy

Hydrotherapy utilizes water to treat the body and mind. Its aim is to bring back health using water-based methods including steam baths, cold compresses, and steam. It is widely believed Hydrotherapy was invented through the work of father Sebastian Kneipp, who was monk of the 19th century. He believed that illnesses could be treated through the use of water to flush out bodily waste. There's a science that explains Hydrotherapy in which the cold (chilled waters) can enlarge blood vessels and thus increase circulation of blood to organs. However warmth (hot water) can eliminate metabolic waste from the body. Thus changing between cold and hot water, like numerous Hydrotherapy treatments do, could decrease inflammation, improve circulation, and improve your health.

Here are a few of the therapies that could be provided during a hydrotherapy session:

Sitz bath. The patient puts his feet in a tub of water before sitting on the other. One bathtub is filled with cool water, the second is hot. The patient then switches places to alternate between heated and cold pools.

Wraps. Sheets that have been submerged with cold water can be placed around the patient when lying on. The blanket is then surrounded with dry towels and blankets. The body will naturally heat up to fight the chill.

This helps to treat inflammation and pain in the muscles and many other health problems.

Hot water soaks. The patient is soaked with warm, warm water up to an hour. Different ingredients are put into the water including oils or muds, as well as sea salts.

Sauna. The patient lies in a sauna that is flooded with dry warm.

Massage Therapy

Massage Therapy is among the most sought-after Naturopathic treatments. It not only helps patients unwind and relax, it can also help with certain ailments and improve wellbeing. When you go through a typical massage the practitioner uses specific movements to give the body and mind with various advantages. There are many kinds of massages available, each one having distinct advantages. For instance, although Swedish massages are great to relax, those who suffer from joint pain might be able to benefit from Shiatsu treatments are beneficial.

The kind of massage you choose to use will be based on your individual preferences and conditions. It's generally recommended to test various types of massage to determine what works the best for your situation.

In order to give you a clear picture of what each technique includes (so you can select the one that is most effective for you) I've provided an explanation of the most commonly used kinds of massages used in the present:

Swedish massages are usually the first thing that come into your mind when you think of massage. The massage is comprised of deliberate, slow moves that ease muscles, ease tension, and soothe the body, mind, and soul. The client is generally instructed to remove her clothing and drape herself in a sheet so that she doesn't get visible during the treatment. A light lotion, cream or oil is applied by the practitioner during the massage. The session generally lasts around an hour. But, you are able to schedule shorter or longer sessions as needed. Swedish massage is comprised of four main actions: effleurage and friction as well as tapotement. Effleurage is comprised of lengthy slow strokes. Petrissage involves kneading the muscle and tissue. Friction moves boost circulation and warm the muscle tissue.

Likewise, tapotement uses quick-hitting strokes to can tone muscles.

Shiatsu massages are a tradition that originated within the Far East, and has been practiced for many long periods of time. In a Shiatsu massage the client is fully clothed , and the practitioner applies the pressure of the fingers instead of moving in a fluid manner. Shiatsu massages are based on the notion that all of us have meridians of energy (channels) running through our bodies. A Shiatsu massage practitioner will hold and press certain points along these meridians the hope of restoring harmony to your energy flow as well as eliminate any blockages that might be affecting the energy channel.

Deep Tissue massages generally employ various techniques used in Swedish massages, but in addition to other techniques that are designed to penetrate deeper into the muscles and tissues. The main purpose of deep tissue massages is to eliminate tension and knots. Certain movements involve massaging the muscles in a cross-fiber manner and relieves tension kept in muscle tissues and helps eliminate the amount of toxins.

Hot Stone massages typically consist of Swedish massage movements , while hot stones are placed on different parts of the body. Although some massage professionals prefer to apply the stones at strategically placed points on the body (such for the side of the spine or on the back of the legs) and then employ their hands to perform the massage techniques, other practitioners use hot stones in their hands , and apply them to the patient. Massages with hot stones can ease tight muscles and boost circulation.

Lomi Lomi is a more quick form of massage that includes quick, deliberate, and lengthy strokes executed by the therapist's arms instead of the hands. The practice began in Hawaii and is rapidly becoming a popular form of massage therapy because it eases tension and strengthens the muscles.

Trigger Point massages an alternative therapy, which means they're usually performed alongside another type of massage. When used as a stand-alone the type of massage can result in muscle strain. A trigger point massage therapist will locate specific areas of tensed muscles tissues, which are typically identified with an adhesion (commonly known as knot). The therapist then presses down with a firm pressure on the trigger point to ease the tension that will relieve the pressure stored in the muscle group.

The Craniosacral Therapy only addresses the head and is based on the notion that the cerebrospinal liquid that is a part of our brains and spinal cords generates a pulse inside our bodies. The pulse can be detected by the practitioner by placing his hands over your head. The intensity and frequency of the pulse will indicate to the practitioner that there is a problem or problems can be addressed by simply changing the skull's plates.

Massage is a wonderful method of stress reduction. I've been practicing the art of massage for long number of years and am pleased to have helped many people unwind, relax and change their lives through massage. Although some people may consider it an exercise in relaxation but I am able to claim that it is able to improve your health physically as well as emotionally.

Homeopathy

Homeopathy makes use of highly diluted substances to increase the body's healing powers. The first Homeopathic practitioner to be recognized is Samuel Hahnemann, who introduced the method in 1796. The principal theory for this holistic approach to healing is that a substance which creates specific symptoms when consumed in large doses could help treat these symptoms. This is accomplished by providing the patient with smaller doses that are more dilute of the drug. Although homeopathic physicians can prescribe medicines like Ritalin however, their prescriptions are so weak that they can lose a good majority of, if not all of their toxic effects. Thus, patients are able to enjoy the benefits of the drug without worrying about potentially dangerous adverse reactions that might be experienced if they consume more doses.

There are three fundamental principles frequently associated with Homeopathy. Every single remedy which are recommended by Homeopathic doctors is based on the following fundamental theories:

Like cures like. The principle behind Homeopathy is that you can treat similar conditions by taking similar. If, for instance, you have a troubled sleeping pattern, applying a Homeopathic remedy which is known to cause insomnia, like one with caffeine can help you take a rest that you desperately need. This is based on the idea that if a chemical typically produces specific symptoms, it could be reduced and utilized as a remedy which can be used to treat the similar symptoms.

Similar cures alike is called"the "law of likes". Thus, if a health person experiences exposure to a specific substance and suffers symptoms due to it an herbal remedy using the same ingredient can benefit sufferers with identical symptoms though they don't have the condition which the remedy is usually employed to treat.

Give the minimum dose. The homeopathic remedy administered to patients must be as minimally diluted as it is. Most often, the remedy which is given is highly diluted so that you can enjoy all the benefits of the remedy, without being able to experience any side consequences. This is based on the principle of "Potentization" which all homeopathic remedies must follow. The process of potentization is typically quite complex and involves many steps in order to create the most efficient remedy.

Potentization allows patients to reap the benefits of the very low dose of a specific chemical. Additionally, it gives them the possibility of consuming the remedies they choose without worrying about the risk of taking them due to the process of dilution removes contaminants and chemical toxicity which were present in the substance in question. In this way, patients can also help or treat illnesses with substances that would not be suitable for consumption by humans.

Rely on a Single Treatment. Whatever symptoms a patient might be experiencing, they will be offered one treatment at one time. The one remedy is intended to treat the source of the issue as well as every symptom. This is very different from how conventional doctors treat diseases nowadays. For instance, if you see the general practitioner to treat an illness with many distinct symptoms, he may possibly prescribe a medicine to treat each sign that you're experiencing. However, a practitioner of Homeopathy will only prescribe one treatment that is employed to treat all the symptoms associated with your illness and also the root cause of your issue.

It is also crucial to remember that homeopathic remedies can be found in various methods. The method of administration that your holistic doctor decides to use is dependent on your personal preferences, and the ingredients that are used to make the cure. The most popular forms of remedies are available in are gels, creams tablets, pellets, and liquids. Below is some details about each of them:

Tablets. This type of homeopathic treatment is generally soft and is made up of the sugar of milk (known by the name lactose). It is a great choice for children and babies as well as those with difficulty swallowing as it is more digestible and dissolves faster.

Liquids. These remedies are consumed orallyand are extremely potent and powerful. It is generally advised to put off for about an hour before you clean your teeth and then for a half hour before you drink or eat anything when you have taken oral forms of remedies that are homeopathic.

Creams/Gels. This kind of holistic treatment typically is less potent and is not meant to be consumed. Instead, you'll often apply the products on the skin (on your face) to treat any external symptoms.

Pellets. The remedy can be consumed orally and is generally put under one's tongue in which it slowly dissolves. Pellets may be crushed, or dissolve in a glass filled with water.

Iridology

Iridology is a comprehensive examination of the eye of a patient to determine if there are any health issues in the body. In essence, the structures and patterns that make up the eye are studied to ensure that the doctor is able to identify areas that suggest the presence of inflammation in the the body. Although many people believe that the iris is just a color that is influenced by genetics, Iridologists are of the opinion that the iris could tell us something about our body's structure, strengths and weaknesses and the effect of our decisions about our lives.

Iridology's history is an interesting and fascinating one. It was created in the 19th century by Ignatz Von Peczely who was a doctor in the 18th century. As a young child, Ignatz was in his garden when he observed an owl tear its leg in the course of fighting. He ran over towards the injured bird, and noticed that the owl's eye was black. the eye of the owl. While he nursed the injured owl back to health it inspected its eyes and observed as it changed. Later in his life he would claim the direct connection between changes in the body in the eyes and the shape of our eyes.

Iridology is based on the notion that the person's constitution can be assessed through the pattern, fibres, structures as well as the colors and brightness in the eyes. It is also able to tell whether a person suffers from high levels of toxicity or any other dietary issues. When looking at an Iris map or chart The doctor will then provide the patient with information on what body part might require improvement or treated.

Flower Essences

Although flower essence therapies are frequently confused with Aromatherapy It is an entirely different approach. Flower essence therapy is the blossoms of the plant are put into the form of a bowl filled with water and the sun's rays are used to make an infusion. The mixture is then dilute to make it stronger and is preserved using alcohol (usually brandy). It takes a lot of preparation to ensure that the blend is infused with the energy of the flower employed. The belief is that the energy sources assist the body in healing itself and the various essences are able to produce different outcomes.

Therapy using flower essences was developed in the late the Dr. Edward Bach, who was a famous English surgeon. The Dr. Bach believed that there is a direct connection between our emotions and our physical health. The first flower remedies, which were suggested by Dr. Bach, of which there are 38 total were utilized to address the emotional causes of physical ailments. Many people today depend on the use of flower essences to treat medical issues as well as as preventative treatments.

Typically flowers are administered by mouth and then placed on the tongue of the patient. Just a few drops essence is typically all that is needed. You could also add the essence to a glass of water and consume it throughout the day. The various combination of essences could also be utilized to gain various advantages.

Here are some examples of Bach Flower remedies that can be utilized:

Heather is a great way to decrease self-centeredness and increase compassion for other people. It's also a great option for those looking to be better listeners.

Centaury can be used to aid people who have difficulty saying "no" to anyone else. It boosts confidence and self-esteem.

Olive can help to restore energy. It is a great option to help those who feel like they have lost their energy.

Wild Oat enhances our mental concentration and clarity that allows us to remain focused and live out our ultimate goal in life.

Cerato assists us in not be unsure of our own choices and judgements, as well as to trust our own sense of intuition.

Impatience allows the ability to have patience with other people and also to be more calm and considerate when making decisions.

Lifestyle Consultations

A lot of Naturopathic doctors use Lifestyle Consultations to offer their patients with a comprehensive treatment plan. They'll inquire what you are eating, exercises, and any other lifestyle choices which could have an immediate influence on your mental or physical well-being. They could also suggest modifications that you can implement to your routine or provide you with a couple of tips you can utilize to boost your overall health. A Lifestyle Consultant will give you suggestions to improve almost all aspects of life. This will improve your mood as well.

Chapter 4: The Benefits Of Naturopathy

There are many advantages you can anticipate to get from regular Naturopathic therapies. It's crucial to remember that the outcomes of Naturopathy will differ significantly between patients and are largely dependent on your personal medical condition and the treatment you decide to use. Although one patient may discover that Naturopathy can significantly help with their ailments while another may find that the Naturopathic treatments they choose to use can provide peace and improved emotional wellbeing. But, there are some benefits that have been well-documented or have been published. Here are some of the advantages of Naturopathy treatments:

The goal is to address the root of the problem, rather than just treating symptoms. This could speed up the healing process and may keep the illness from recurring in future instances.

Don't rely on prescription drugs or medications to treat your health issue. So, you don't need to worry about the side reactions or potentially harmful adverse reactions that some people suffer from when they take medication.

It can be utilized to maintain your health after your medical condition is resolved. In the end, it will improve your overall health and improve your quality of your life.

The doctor will consider the whole patient's overall health status, not only the present ailment. So, your mental and emotional health is assessed and assisted not solely your physical health.

It is safe for both children and older adults, as opposed to other types of treatment. Thus, nearly everybody will gain of Naturopathy in some manner shape, manner, or.

Every treatment plan provided by a Naturopath is individualized to the individual patient. The practitioner uses the combination of a range of treatments and methods that include herbal medicine along with nutritional consultations and massage therapy to address the problem. This means that every patient will reap the greatest benefits from their treatment.

The treatment of conditions that conventional medical treatment cannot. For instance in the event that a patient suffering from a severe medical condition, medicines might not offer the greatest benefit, but the use of chiropractic or flower essence therapy can significantly improve their overall health.

If you're looking for a natural method of healing, then Naturopathy could be the best alternative. A Naturopathic Practitioner can treat your medical problem conducting a variety of tests including the blood test as well as a comprehensive medical history analysis to provide an accurate picture of the overall condition of your health. She will then be able to identify the illness you're suffering from and help you restore your health with the use of all-natural treatments. You may also decide to consult a Naturopath once you're in good health, to ensure that you can maintain your healthy balance in your body and your mind.

Health Conditions that may benefit from Naturopathy

Although almost all people is able to benefit from Naturopathy however, there are some ailments that could be greatly improved with Naturopathic treatments. Because Naturopathy doesn't cause negative unwanted side effects it is very rare to find diseases or conditions that can't be treated in some way through Naturopathic treatments.

Here are some of the illnesses that Naturopathy might be able to relieve or completely treat:

Allergic reactions (seasonal or food allergy can be cured)

Arthritis, and other conditions that cause inflammation

Depression

Anxiety

The chronic backache

Chronic Fatigue Syndrome

- Joint pain

Thrush (Candida)

The blood pressure of high pressure

Irritable Bowel Syndrome

- Insomnia and sleep problems

Migraines

Elbow Tennis Elbow

The most common cause is Poly Cystic Ovarian Syndrome

- Menopause

- Endometriosis

Prostate - Larger Prostate

- Skin conditions

- Problems with weight

- Fibromyalgia

- Medical conditions related to age

- Immunity - Deficiencies

Constipation

Ulcers

Remember that these are only one of the many illnesses that can be addressed by Naturopathy. If you suffer from a condition not on the list, it might be beneficial to consult an accredited Naturopath in your region to determine whether Naturopathic treatments might be beneficial. Because no medication or procedures that are invasive are used in the treatment process, Naturopathy is often an option for those who aren't the best candidates for conventional medical treatments. It is so numerous treatments that fall within the umbrella called "naturopathy" and patients will surely find the method or technique that is most suitable for their specific medical needs.

Tips for Naturopathy

It is recommended to seek help with a certified Naturopath however, there are many ways you can start incorporating Naturopathic concepts into your everyday routine. This will help increase the efficacy of your treatments, and provide you the capacity to maximize the benefits of your day and get rid of your illness faster. A lot of the holistic healing practices you'll discover here aren't too complicated or difficult to understand. Actually, many of them are easy and easy tips that will significantly assist you in attaining an enlightened mental and physical body.

Start your day by chanting a positive mantra. When you first wake up, you should take just a few moments to kick your day with a positive attitude. Make yourself feel like you are having the most enjoyable day you can by repeating a positive affirmation for example, "This day is going to be awesome and filled with positivity and I'm capable of making any thing happen". This can help improve your mood and help you get your thoughts moving toward the correct direction throughout your day. Thinking positive thoughts will release powerful chemicals into our brains, which improve our overall wellbeing, including serotonin.

Exercise. Maintaining a healthy lifestyle and making sure you do sufficient exercise is among the easiest ways to boost your overall health. When you have time free from work, you should try to go outside and take in the outdoors. Take a walk, run, or perhaps spend the day at the beach or in the park. This will allow you to exercise while enjoying yourself and being with family and your friends. If you are working, ensure that you have frequent breaks in order to move through the area and move. A long time at work can reduce the flow of blood and lymph and can hamper your efforts to keep balance. If you're unable to get yourself out of the office to exercise simply spend a few minutes to practice some yoga exercises at your desk or stretch your arms while performing certain breathing techniques.

Have an Naturopathic Shower. Before you get in the shower make use of a loofah that is dry to massage your skin. Create small, gentle circles that start at your feet and move toward your neck. This will help to clean off dead skin cells and increase circulation. It also improves the flow of blood through the heart, and can even help reduce varicose veins as well as the possibility of blood clots. Your lymph system is also likely to benefit from this method, considering that dry brushing may allow for wastes and toxins to be flushed out your body more rapidly. After you have finished dry brushing (which will take only one or two minutes) take a trip to the shower and bathe like you would normally. Before leaving take the time to finish your shower by increasing the temperature of the water for around 60 seconds and then turning the temperature down to cold for another minute or more. Repeat this process three to four times in succession. This is referred to as"a "contrast shower" which will increase the circulation of your body and eliminate toxic substances that can cause health issues.

Pay attention to what you consume. There's a saying that goes: "you are what you consume". Although it's an old fashioned saying, it's 100% true. Every food you consume has an impact on your health and mood. It is important to take a healthy breakfast every day and take healthy snacks whenever you leave your house for work. Consuming small portions of healthy food throughout the day can boost your energy levels and boost your metabolism. Fruits and nuts make excellent snack options for on the go.

Create a peaceful sleeping environment. It is essential to can create the best sleeping space within your room. Decorate it in a way that creates the feeling of a peaceful space. Paint it with soothing colors when painting your walls, or select serene pieces of art. Try to avoid making use of your space for activities other than sleep like office work. If you do have a workstation in the bedroom make sure to cover it during the time of night or split the space into different sections with an area partition. Ideally, you'd like to create a space within your home in which you are relaxed and at peace, so you can have a more peaceful sleep. Also, make sure that you ensure that your space is clear of clutter and rest in complete darkness. This will allow you to regulate your sleeping patterns and improve your overall well-being.

Keep a Naturopath Journal. Note down what you're experiencing every day, and any other information regarding your life that you think is essential. This will allow you to examine your feelings and track your daily routine. It is also possible to add a section on eating as well as a mood section within your daily journal and also the physical activities you take part in. This will enable you to discern a link between your exercise and eating habits as well as your mood.

Pay attention to your breathing. Check your breathing all day long. Most of the time, you'll notice that you're not taking deep breaths as you should. In reality, you may even find that your breathing is slow and shallow. This is due to the fact that we don't concentrate and be aware of our breathing. Take deep breaths into and out slowly to increase the amount of oxygen you are getting.

Make time to think about your day. After each day spend a few minutes to think about what transpired and try to find some positive aspect to concentrate on. Make sure you are grateful for the good things that happen in your life and do your best to not allow the negative thoughts to stop you from feeling optimistic about the future.

Include aromatherapy in your daily routines. While you go through your day, you should try to include aromatherapy in your daily routine whenever you can. It will help you enjoy the benefits of aromatherapy, such as peace, improved well-being as well as increased energy levels, as well as an improvement in your immune system depending on the oil you select. You can light a candle in your office or at home. utilize a car air freshener or apply a small amount your preferred essential oil for inhaling the scent all day long.

Chapter 5: Faq About Naturopathy

What exactly is Naturopathic Medicine, and how is it different with traditional medicines?

Naturopathic Medicine is a way to find the root of the disease or ailment instead of just managing the symptoms it creates. It can also improve your general well-being and improve your physical and mental health. Instead of asking about the factors the cause of your specific health problem, Naturopaths attempt to determine why you're experiencing the problem even. They will concentrate on the whole patient.

The primary distinction between the Naturopathic practitioner and conventional medical doctor is that a Naturopathic doctor will examine the lifestyle choices, the emotional well-being, as well as physical health of an individual and not only the effects of the condition they suffer from. They then employ remedies and natural methods to address the issue and avoid medication or invasive procedures.

What types of treatments are available? Naturopaths usually provide?

The therapies provided by Naturopaths differ greatly based on the practitioner you select. However, Naturopaths generally utilize a variety of strategies in treating patients. This is because the majority of Naturopathic treatments are based on the same fundamental principles and principles. Fundamentally, Naturopathy is all about healing the body itself through a little stimulation. Examples that Naturopathic treatments that can be provided are: manipulation of the body, Traditional Chinese Medicine, massage, and other treatments.

Are Naturopathy insured by insurance? If so, and most importantly is it safe?

Since some Naturopathy treatments are considered "new" by certain insurance providers, you might discover that your insurance provider will not cover your Naturopathy treatments. However, it is suggested that you contact your insurance provider to find out if they cover your specific treatments. If you have spend money out of your pocket you'll discover that Naturopathy is usually worthwhile for every dollar. It is because you get an ability to recover yourself without the use of expensive medicines or surgical procedures that take an extensive amount of recovery time.

Concerning the security of Naturopathy The treatments that are employed are typically non-invasive, gentle and completely natural. So there is a low chance of experiencing negative side effects that are that are associated with the Naturopathic methods. This means that it is suitable for everyone of all ages.

What can I expect from an average Naturopathy appointment?

The appointment you make with a Naturopathic doctor will be contingent on your plan of treatment and the doctor that you decide to decide to choose. The initial appointment typically includes a thorough examination of your current state of health along with a range of tests. For instance, many physicians conduct lab tests and tests during your first visit. They can also ask you specific questions regarding your diet and lifestyle.

Chapter 6: The Philosophy Behind

Naturopathy

A few people consider naturopathy "the art of living" and live their lives based on the fundamental concepts of this discipline. This is because naturopathy does not intend to just provide an alternative treatment to ailments. It is designed to provide rehabilitation of the mind, body as well as the soul. Naturopathy advocates say that you can't be well if one or more of the elements are not pure. So, it is essential to be at peace with yourself and the environment around you in order in order to reach the fullest extent.

Modern medicine often ignores the vitality of our bodies. This energy is our primary allies when we wish to make a change in our life and be happy and healthy. People who choose natural healing as a method to live do not simply abandon modern medications and change everything they do. Their diet, their views on the world around them and their commitment to living an active and healthy life are transformed. If one eliminates the negative aspects which surround them, they have more room to focus on positive energy.

The power of the mind and spirit is an essential component of healing for any illness or injury. The body is also affected not just by external influences like the environment and food sources, but as well by negative thoughts and energy emanating from the inside. When a person experiences bad news or becomes angry, the individual may begin to feel sick physically due to emotions can have a huge influence in our wellbeing. In order to ensure the proper functioning of the body, it's essential to avoid negative thoughts and to understand how to manage your emotions. If a person gets angry and often caused by circumstances beyond their control, the person is causing harm to the body as well as the spirit. However, when one is in total control of their thoughts the health begins to improve dramatically.

The concept of emotion affecting your health is something healers have been aware of for years and is now something that modern medicine accepts. If you're happy your body will take care of itself. Most doctors will employ as a last resort"the "Placebo effect" for patients. In this method, doctors will administer fake medications and make patients believe that they can assist them in becoming healthy. In reality, the majority of these patients actually become healthy. Patients suffering from severe illness, such as cancer or other fatal illnesses recover in a span of a mere few months, thanks to this technique called the Placebo Effect. These "magical" recuperations are evidence that by utilizing positivity and the strength of the spirit individuals can tackle problems that appear impossible to solve. However, many people get caught up in a surface world, where everything has an emotional reaction that they forget that we are more than just the bones and flesh.

The body's energy makes people achieve amazing feats. The case that brought naturopathy into the public's notice was a tragic accident within the United States several years ago. A mother saw her child being sucked under the car, and was able to free the vehicle - that weighed 2,000 pounds - by herself. Scientists have said that this was caused by an overdose of adrenaline. But this just confirms the basic concept of

Naturopathy. We are blessed with a power that we don't know what to do with it.

A lot of people believe that naturopathic physicians are health experts who study old books and get their knowledge from mythology. They actually study the same fundamental sciences as conventional doctors however they adopt an alternative approach, believing that the importance of prevention over treating. Naturopathy isn't the same as what mainstream media portrays intentionally or unintentionally, only about using herbal remedies and meditation to cure a common cold. The majority of treatments made with natural medicine are recognized, if not explicitly prescribed by modern medical professionals. The difference between these two is the fact that modern medicine utilizes ingredients that are processed so thoroughly that they lose their benefits, whereas natural medicine utilizes the identical ingredients in their natural form.

If doctors suggest that patients rest or avoids food processed and consumes lots of liquids and drinks without knowing it that the doctor is recommending natural remedies. A balanced, healthy lifestyle is what is needed to get rid of the majority of diseases, not many new remedies. It's more sensible to stop an illness from developing than treat each one once it has a chance to manifest. Of course, it is possible to use a medication to alleviate headaches, but it does not identify or address the root reason for the discomfort. This means that the issue continues to arise until the individual becomes dependent on medications.

There are a variety of treatments that are that are used as alternative medicines, all having proven effective in addressing specific problems that people are likely to face. Physical activities, meditation and a diet that is vegan are all part of naturopathy. they all help to strengthen or restore natural defense systems, while preserving the natural balance of chemicals in the body.

Many people are hesitant when they first attempt to make use of the practice of naturopathy. It's a little absurd that plants and meditation can treat ailments that were too complex in the modern world of medicine handle. One principle is the basis of all the beliefs behind the practice of naturopathy, which is that We are equipped with all the tools we require to combat any illness in our own. The body is made to heal itself, however the body's natural healing processes can do this only if in a safe environment. If we choose to take pills that are laden in hidden poisons, we block the natural healing processes and alter the chemical makeup that our bodies have. The fact that the rate of death from illnesses are rising each year indicates that modern medicine is failing. If these toxic drugs were as effective as they appear to be, the death rates would fall and we'd have less sick patients each year. An objective look at the present situation shows that we must return to our roots and utilize the resources we've always utilized.

the benefits of naturalopathy

There are numerous advantages of naturopathy. However, we will highlight the most well-known and significant ones.

In the beginning, naturopathy is a remedy for the spirit and soul. It's not just another medicine that can relieve your headaches, but it could be among the most effective ways you live your life. When people began applying naturalopathic principles realized how each day their lives were transformed. Beyond the benefits of a well-balanced blood pressure and pain management this lifestyle change altered their outlook on life. A different way of living could result in improvement in each and every aspect that you were unhappy with or was causing you discomfort. It also can bring peace and tranquility that nothing other form of treatment or therapy will bring. As an example, many doctors suggest natural remedies for those suffering from depression severe because it takes more than just a couple of pills to restore the spirit.

In addition, naturopathy may increase the body's ability to regenerate by opening the flow of energy which is blocked by the decades of modern-day aliments and busy schedules. If you are suddenly suffering from migraines or pain, it's not because you didn't get enough rest. It's because your body, mind and your soul aren't in perfect harmony. You need to find balance in your life. When you apply the holistic approach to your daily life, your relationships with other people are bound to improve drastically. A person who is content and has positive energy can be an attraction for those seeking a break from their hectic lives.

The third, and possibly most important benefit of the practice of naturopathy is that it keeps your body from the harmful substances used in medical treatments. Chemicals, regardless of whether they are intended to help you heal in the long run, always create unbalance in chemical makeup of your body. It could cause more harm than beneficial in the end. Additionally, when you take many medications, you may be at a higher chance of developing depression and anxiety since many of them interfere with your body's natural endorphin production, which is the chemical that help us feel happy.

If you're looking for efficient solutions for your medical condition, you'll be pleased to know that naturopathy has the ability in the treatment of many ailments that modern medicine is able to only alleviate. There are a few instances when natural remedies have been utilized effectively in challenging situations for patients who are terminal or those with cancerous tumors that are dangerous to their health. But, the majority of people utilize natural remedies to treat simpler problems like ailment of stomach or insomnia. Numerous simple treatments, such as herbal infusions and homeopathy could solve these medical issues without the use of chemicals.

Additionally, many skin conditions are treated through Acupuncture or using natural lotions. The creams and lotions recommended by physicians are made in natural components. But these products lose their healing qualities when they are made, as the ingredients that are active are insignificant in what is created. If you are looking for a cosmetic treatment, it's better to replace the current cosmetics with organic alternatives. They will not only help you look younger but also keep you healthy and give your skin the supplements that it requires to shine.

In the end, there are few ailments that naturopathy can't treat. With the exception of those that require surgical intervention the body has all the necessary resources to be able to heal and function normally. The only thing we need to do is learn how to utilize them , and be living our lives to our fullest capacity.

Natural Treatments

Yoga

Yoga is among the best methods to control your mind, body and soul. It's actually the solution to many of the problems that we confront every day. Many consider it to be an artform, while others engage in it as a form of sport, while others just want to experience the tranquil benefits of the meditation that goes along in the process. It was originally a practice of the ancient, Indian art is now one of the most popular ways to heal spiritually.

The practice of Yoga helps your body, mind as well as your spirit. It is believed by Naturopaths to be the best method to heal and prevent ailments. It is among the best ways of improving mental stability is the meditative aspect of Yoga has been a blessing to many who were suffering from ailments that traditional medicine could do nothing to help. Yoga helps people to remain in total harmony with the surrounding world by connecting their most profound thoughts. As they discover and direct the body's natural energy individuals can experience a brand completely new and exciting world in which they control everything. The individual is not in control of the events that happen to them, however, they have total control of the way they respond to it. You can't make your boss more tolerant however, you can alter the way that someone's behavior influences your mood, If you're in charge of your emotions.

Yoga is a multifaceted science that covers a wide range of physical and mental well-being. A regular practice can lead to an improved balance in life. It can also lead to an alteration in one's diet. A lot of people who practice yoga eventually go vegetarian. One of the fundamental tenets of yoga and Naturopathy generally is that to stay healthy, it is essential to eat a diet based with natural, unprocessed foods. Yoga enthusiasts, those who are those who practice Yoga typically consider eating animal products to be absorbing negative energy which could cause an imbalance to the body. Even those who consume meat products are of the opinion that refined modern diet is among the major factors that cause the majority of ailments.

"Asanas" are particular Yoga positions that, used in conjunction with a concentrated breathing technique and meditation, provide healing benefits that offer a range of health benefits to your body. Insomnia, depressionand indigestion and muscle pains resulting from an insufficient immune system are all able to be treated and prevented by the most basic postures of Yoga. Most doctors would recommend chemical remedies for these signs however, they are not necessary. The majority of the time, these bio imbalances are merely an indication that we're not in good health, that we are eating poorly or are over-stressing ourselves with trivial things. Any illness that isn't the result of an imbalance in chemical balance cannot be resolved by a high dose of chemicals.

One of the key elements of Yoga is breathing techniques. Simply by controlling your enthusiasm and exhalation, you can ease your body, ease your pain and assist in reducing insomnia. There are a variety of breathing techniques, each is appropriate to a particular Yoga posture. The general rule is that anyone will benefit from this method. You can use it wherever and anytime you'd like.

Acupuncture

Acupuncture is now widely utilized in the cosmetic industry. Alongside its health benefits, the people became aware of the practice after scientists discovered the incredible effects this treatment could provide to the skin. Many patients are using this treatment in order to maintain their complexion looking young and smooth.

Acupuncture employs a holistic approach to heal illnesses that are prevalent in the present. Its roots are in ancient China and is widely used as a substitute for conventional medicine. The concept behind acupuncture focuses on 12 meridian channels, and two central channels which send energy throughout the body. If the channel is blocked obstruction and energy flows are blocked, these rivers do not flow in a normal manner and disruptions to the normal functioning of the body occur. The energy that is blocked is known as "Chi" by practitioners of acupuncture. it is utilized to relieve pain, relieve tension or stress, and to heal damaged skin.

The process of acupuncture involves the placement of tiny needles to the skin on key points. This procedure restores energy balance, and encourages your body to utilize its healing powers in the most needed regions. Patients who were not diagnosed by a conventional doctor got their answers through acupuncture experts. Energy channels aren't accepted as real in medical profession of today. A specialist in acupuncture can identify and correct the imbalance that causes the symptoms. Someone who is suffering from insomnia and is taking medications for years with no success may see relief after just one or two sessions of Acupuncture. Even though the placement of needles may be intimidating at first there isn't any discomfort or pain.

There are many variations of Acupuncture, where the physician uses electrical or heat at specific areas. The electrical stimulation is typically utilized for facial treatments and it is currently an effective treatment to treat the appearance of wrinkles, scars and lines. The stimulation of the skin with electricity causes the skin to make collagen it is the type of protein which provides the skin elasticity.

Acupuncture therapy is also used all over the world to treat muscle pain. The needle being inserted at a specific location of the muscle will relieve tension and will relieve the pain nearly immediately. The use of chemical lotions or pills can treat symptoms however they will not address the root of the problem. Acupuncture, on the other hand, will address the root of the problem and help prevent the occurrence of future illnesses.

Modern medical science has accepted Acupuncture as a legitimate medical practice. Currently, doctors are receiving training in this area. It is, however, an approach that has been practiced for many thousands of years and is among the most effective methods of alternative medical practices.

Color Therapy

If you are looking to look for alternative solutions to their issues the use of color therapy has proved to be a viable alternative treatment, particularly for children. A lot of people have observed for a long time, how a specific color that is used on wall surfaces in the bedrooms can help to improve sleeping.

However, the concept of complete color therapy was developed just recently.

Color therapy is among the easiest methods to treat illnesses that require medical treatment. From digestive issues to sleep issues, the effects of a specific color can affect your mood and body. Psychologists have discovered that chromotherapy can be beneficial, particularly for children who have Autism or Attention Deficit Hyperactivity Disorder or as a type treatment for cognitive disorders. Chromotherapists claim that employing different colors, we can actually regulate the energy levels in our bodyand are able to compensate for what are lacking. Researchers have studied the subject and have found out that using certain colors could cause some hormones within the brain, altering our mood and reducing discomfort.

Utilizing colors to affect the mood is now able to be utilized extensively for interior designs. Designers have realized the effect the color of a room can have on people , and how a particular color on a wall can create the distinction between a kitchen that is normal or one that stimulates your appetite. Restaurants, bars and shops all make use of the power of color to create emotions and feelings and affect the customers. Often, you will observe how a particular hue instantly can make you feel happy, or sad.

Color therapy is accessible to everyone It is not necessary to require any prior training or a lot of knowledge to use it. All you have to do is inform yourself of the impact of various colors and using that knowledge you can make improvements to your life in general.

Colors don't just have an effects on our moods as well as our physical bodies. Blood pressure can be elevated or decreased by the use of blue and red. The digestion can be improved by applying the color green to the food areas and also we can get an enjoyable night's sleep in our bedroom if it is decorated in dark shades such as brown or burgundy.

Photobiology The scientific study of the effects of various lighting and colors on living organisms, was created in the wake of the introduction the concept of color therapy. While modern science does not entirely accept the relationship between medical treatments and colors however, certain scientists admit that it may trigger an uplifting response to patients who are exposed to various kinds of light.

Reiki

Human beings, as a species are composed of more than just flesh and bones. We have an inner strength and power that naturalists are focused on. Although modern medicine claims to provide answers to our questions, it isn't the case. Modern medicine isn't the solution, instead, it's an approach to treat the symptoms. If we're suffering from illness, we suffer in a deeper way and in the very core of our being.

Reiki is a practice that has been around for a long time which was revived recently by those who believe we are able of healing ourselves. The Reiki concept is based on the energy points of our body , referred to as "chakras." The chakras are situated within our endocrine glands, and, when combined, create the invisible field of energy that surrounds us. It is possible to receive and transmit energy to the living creatures all around us, from animals to humans. The Reiki practitioner believes that when the energy source gets damaged or something is preventing an energy flow we suffer on both a mental as well as physical level.

In the same way, every person has the capacity to heal this energy as well as to help others. But, the majority of people don't use this ability, and are lost between when they reach adulthood and childhood. It is the Reiki instructors have either maintained or even regained this power and are able to help others learn how to harness their own energy to assist others. Through opening every chakra as well as teaching to focus your energy, you'll be able to transmit positive energy to your fingers.

Anyone who chooses to do Reiki are also pledging to transform their lives positively. They try to stay away from negative thoughts, master the art of attracting positive energy and learn to feel content with their lives. This helps to live a happy and peaceful life that is that is in harmony with the world that surrounds you. When someone gets sick, it's due to the fact that an energy point is affected by external forces. This means that whenever negative energies are greater than positive ones and there are negative health effects. Reiki practitioners Reiki practitioner is able to use the positive energies of his clients to help heal us and assist us to regain our power. The benefits have been proved for migraines, muscular pain and insomnia, digestive disorders and depression. Certain skin conditions can be treated using internal energy. If you live an active, stressful life, this kind of therapy could be the ideal solution to avoid various health issues.

Homeopathy

Homeopathy is a form of holistic medicine that is based on the idea that we must treat the patient and not just the illness. It first came into use during the 1800s and is currently widely recommended by a growing number of physicians as an alternative treatment.

This kind of therapy utilizes the natural capacity that the body has to recover itself. There are two methods to heal - the same and the opposite. Homeopathy follows the same method and this means that a homeopath physician will prescribe small amounts of caffeine that are administered in a manner that will result in the opposite effect anticipated.

The drugs that are administered in homeopathic medicines are not addicting, and they are not harmful to the body as they are only prescribed in small amounts. They are not specifically designed to treat illness, but can be used to help stimulate the body to fight the illness. There are a variety of homeopathic remedies that are recommended and prescribed by physicians in various areas. The components were, at the beginning, all natural. However, as homeopathy has spread across the globe, certain remedies are now manufactured in factories.

The homeopathic treatment is now highly sought-after by people suffering from allergies or people who are resistant to modern medications. One of the major aspects that makes homeopathy treatment efficient is the fact that it can be tailored to each patient based on their medical history and personal preferences, such as diet, mode of living, or levels of stress by a personalized medical plan that is developed by a homeopath physician. The homeopath doctor creates your personal treatment plan that is completely tailored to your requirements.

Homeopathy is considered to be, for a lot of people, the most effective alternative to modern medical system. Instead of focusing solely on symptoms, it can prevent the onset of various diseases, instead of attempting to treat the symptoms as they develop. The homeopathic treatments do not alter the chemical balance that is natural to the body. Instead, they help to stimulate the healing process. If we consume a drug with toxic ingredients, we actually alter the body's chemistry and are affecting not just its immunity but also its ability to fight off diseases in the over the long haul.

Ayurvedic Medicine

Ayurvedic Medicine is an ancient practice that was discovered in India hundreds of years ago. it's based on Vedic texts, which are India's sacred texts. It's like other naturopathic branches such as homeopathy or Chinese herbal remedies. However, unlike other remedies that are natural it is an entire system that is based around the practice of meditation Yoga along with a strict regimen of food.

The Ayurvedic life style is founded on harmony in all aspects of our lives, including sleeping, diet sexual relations, emotions and physical exercise. Anyone who chooses to explore Ayurvedic medicine will have to go through an entire plan that has to be followed strictly so that you can achieve the ideal balance between body, mind and soul.

A majority of patients begin by undergoing a thorough detoxification not just physically, but mentally. There are a variety of detoxification regimens, ranging including intermittent fasting and herbal drinks. The practitioners of this practice believe it is essential to cleanse our body and the mind prior to attempting to repair any injuries. Some people even have long-term Water Fasts, ranging between 3 and 4 weeks. During this period they only drink water, and do nothing but light Yoga as well as other forms of meditation. Fasting is an integral part of the practice for all religions around the world, and contemporary medical practices have begun to acknowledge its advantages. The belief is that one week of water Fasting can give your body the chance to channel all energy to healing , and not be occupied with digestive and absorption. After breaking a fast the majority of people will adopt the diet of fruits and vegetables, while reducing or eliminating meat, processed foods.

For those who aren't able to perform Water Fasts, the practitioners of Ayurvedic Medicine recommend juice fasting to flush out toxins and allow the body to rest. This means that for a few days, the person will drink only healthy and freshly-made juices. The people who tried this have reported that they did not have a feeling of hunger, but they have stopped craving food and noticed that they fell asleep less, but were more refreshed.

Aromatherapy

Aromatherapy is regarded as an individual exercise or component of Ayurvedic Medicine. It is usually associated with fasting and meditation and is the use in the form of natural oils, or extracts to provide treatment for various ailments.

There is no doubt that certain scents can have an impact on our mood and can affect our mood all day. Vanilla's subtle scent can help us relax after a long day, and lavender fragrance can aid in getting us to rest more comfortably. But the impact of perfumes on health is still in controversy. The use of essential oils has proven beneficial to those suffering from digestive disorders, insomnia nausea, anxiety, or insomnia. Utilizing essential oils with hot water you will also ease the symptoms of the flu and seasonal allergies.

In conjunction in conjunction with meditation, or Yoga, Aromatherapy has incredible effects on the mental and spiritual. Not only does it help reduce depression, but it may help with a variety of mental afflictions. Practitioners of Ayurvedic Medical or Reiki often include scents during their meditation sessions and they believe that it aids in the flow of energy naturally. Together with Acupuncture can produce amazing pain relief and those who suffer from chronic pain can finally lead the life of a normal person. Aromatherapy is a particular type of therapy that is now used in retail stores and workplaces where scents are utilized to make customers feel relaxed and comfortable.

How To Utilize Naturopathy Your Everyday Life

If you choose to alter your life style and utilize natural substances instead of the chemical alternatives, then there's fundamental steps you must follow and a specific mental attitude you must create. There is no need to be an Yoga expert or conduct regular acupuncture sessions to use the art of naturopathy. You can make small changes that you can make in order to lead an improved, more pleasant life. A lot of people follow the principles of naturopathy without even realizing that they are following a healthy and balanced lifestyle that they avoid rather than treat ailments. A balanced diet, continuous physical exercise and a positive outlook are, at the end of the day natural remedies in themselves. If you want to learn more about the practice of naturopathy, there are plenty of classes you can attend or trained specialists can speak to. In the meantime, there are easy remedies you can use in your daily routine without having to put in a lot of effort.

Insomnia may be probably one of the top frequent sleep disorders in modern times. It is true that hectic and stress-filled lives are the main causes. Instead of saturating yourself with sleeping pills, consider some alternatives that are natural and won't harm your body over the long run, and will allow you the restful sleep you desire. Ashwagandha is a well-known herb well-known for its anti-depressant effects. It is primarily used in the Ayurveda Medicine. When it is taken in small doses prior to sleeping and will put you at ease and can eliminate insomnia. If you're looking for a treatment that doesn't require any type of substance, a brief time of Yoga can be effective. In the absence of any complex postures just sit and meditate in your breathing 15 minutes prior to going to bed. The stress-inducing thoughts will go away instantly, and you'll be able to sleep peacefully and restful sleep.

For a boost in your mood and boost your appetite, attempt to implement the principles of color therapy to your home. Paint the walls of your house in hues that aid you in managing every aspect of your day. For instance, you can paint the walls of your dining area or kitchen in a dark shade to increase appetite and avoid digestive issues. A soothing color in your living space, such as dark brown or beige can create a warm and intimate space and increase your time spent with your loved ones. In your bedroom blue can bring a sense of freshness when you wake up, while the cherry-colored walls will place you into a peaceful, restful sleep. It is also possible to use various objects to create colored areas that can improve your mood throughout the day.

To boost your immunity and to avoid seasonal allergies, make use of a homeopathic remedy which is widely used. Mix 10 teaspoons of honey with 3 teaspoons of the boxthorn. Then put the mixture into an enclosed jar for at least 2 weeks. A small spoonful of this mixture every day will not only boost your energy and boost your digestion, but also increase your immunity and protect your body from suffering from colds during the winter. Furthermore, it will keep your appetite in check during the day and you won't be tempted to snack during meals.

If you are suffering from pimples, acne, or bursts frequently on your skin , and you can't pinpoint the root of the problem the natural ointment that is made of Mezereum could be beneficial. Daphne Mezereum is a plant that has been used from the beginning of time for treating skin disorders or provide a sense of peace to anxious patients. Today, a few modern products contain this herb however, the majority the healing qualities are lost when it comes to manufacturing. Mezereum extract is available in the bio-stores or can make your own ointment yourself and apply it at least once a week to avoid pimples and other skin issues.

Chapter 7: Homeopathy

If you've figured out the foundation of naturopathy, and also that, along with the naturopathic certification you must select the various treatments in which you wish to specialize, it's worthwhile to look into the homeopathic method as an additional certification.

This section explains the history and the major aspects of this fascinating treatment. It was initially created by Dr. Samuel Hahnemann at the end of the 18th century. He was based in Germany Hahnemann was sent to study medicine, but he became dissatisfied by the absence of clinical experience and moved into Vienna where he was able to graduate with honors in 1779. Hahnemann began his medical studies within Saxony but was shocked by the savage treatments that were that were being used at the time, treatment which included amputations and the use of arsenic as well as other poisons.

Hahnemann was extremely outspoken. He soon resentment with colleagues and patients and, as a result that he decided to leave the medical field and became an Chemist. To help the family of his parents, he translated medical texts into German. When he was translating a book from William Cullinan - a Scottish physician - that he became intrigued about the claim about the fact that the bark from the cinchona tree could be beneficial in treating malaria.

Hahnemann experienced firsthand this, but he felt that the claim must be wrong and, therefore, he determined to study and test on the effect of the bark on himself only for him to realize that after a week to two days, the bark caused the symptoms of malaria , however when he taken the bark off the symptoms disappeared.

The time was when physicians believed that the major healing process originated from the patient's body, and that treatments affected or hindered healing. In his experiment with Cinchona bark, he argued that there was a second reason. It is possible that the body's healing response wasn't strong enough by itself, however when you added an artificial disease which was in this case, 'the Cinchona bark', it was evident that the body could respond much more efficiently.

This led to an energy-based model of disease and health. His idea of treating patients with like' remains as a fact today. He thought that when you gave an treatment that could cause symptoms, and then in fact be akin to the actual illness it would increase the ability of the patient to recover faster. It was referred to as homoeopathy and comes in the Greek word that means 'similar treatment'.

Hahnemann continued to study by diluting certain of the most toxic substances, believing that they could be utilized for healing with the proper dosages, and it was possible to test his theories on patients, as the research materials he used included. In the end, Hahnemann relocated to Paris where he was made well-known.

At this point he realized that when the medicine bowls were shaken throughout the process of preparation the potency would increase and this was called the process of potentization. He also realized that when the substances were dispersed more widely and diluted, they also increased their effectiveness.

At the time of his death in 1843, he'd refined his research to ensure that the future practitioners followed an established pattern of conduct that included an interview and examination of the patient in order to identify individual symptoms. And the practitioners would then formulate one dose of treatment to set the healing process into motion. The process was later known as homoeopathy classical. Hanuman was a popular figure and homoeopathy was introduced into the United States where further studies were initiated.

At this point in the study, different treatments were tested, and they all matched Hahnemann's initial findings that the cause of the illness or disease is equally crucial. This came to be known as homoeopathy with a constitutional basis. Homoeopathy was introduced to Europe and gained him large followings and numerous institutions and hospitals as well as an organization to certify.

In time, however homoeopathy began to lose popularity and many medical schools started to shut in the US in the year 1950, it was fewer than 100 homoeopathic doctors practicing within the US. Since the time, homoeopathy has returned to recognition and is now an integral component of British and European medical practice.

Homoeopathic remedies are made by dissolving vegetable, mineral or animal components in alcohol, which creates an'mother' tincture. It is a remedy according to the situation, but it is typically diluted with alcohol, or distillate water. Sometimes, trituration occurs (mixing or decreasing particle size) prior to diluting. The dilation and the potent separation of such remedies are established as standard.

Evaluation

Homoeopathic physicians typically require more time to assess the patient than a conventional physician because all symptoms have to be taken into consideration prior to starting treatment. Hahnemann recommended that a doctor should not interrupt the initial consultation, but be attentive and only ask questions when needed. He believed it was essential to determine the root causes of the symptoms as well as their exact location within the body. Also, the doctor wanted comprehend the feelings experienced and be aware of the causes of pain. To be able to understand this how patients judge their symptoms according to their intensity and frequency.

Homoeopathic practitioners today, begin with a questionnaire, which has to be filled out prior to the appointment.

To determine the correct medications to be prescribed the symptoms and the cause need to be determined. This allows a connection to one of the homoeopathic remedies. In the old homoeopathy patients, they were given only one dosage, but the dosages are different, and most people are instructed to consume the remedy at intervals of 15 min. for up to two hours (if they're suffering from acute symptoms) or take 1 tablet (or two or three pellets) every day if they are suffering from chronic ailments however the dosage should be reduced when symptoms begin to diminish.

The remedy type can be modified if symptoms persist into the next week. It is crucial to make sure that homoeopathic remedies don't get consumed for long periods of time. Certainly when the remedy seems to be ineffective the way it was intended, it must be stopped.

The most common homeopathic remedies are:

Arnica montana (Mountain Daisy)

This is among the most popular remedies, and is effective for breathing problems, physical injuries as well as bruising and pain. People who react positively to Arnica typically feel restless and sleep less well at evening and are likely to become anxious. They might have trouble focusing or refusing to acknowledge that something is wrong.

Belladonna (Deadly Nightshade)

Belladonna is a tangled story of an herb that is poisonous, given that it is employed in cosmetics as a poison and as an intoxicant. In terms of homoeopathy it's effective for people suffering from hands that are cold, feel hot, suffers from colds that cause cough or being ill. Patients tend to be anxious at times, agitated or restless. vivid dreams are associated with insomnia. Belladonna is also utilized for relief from colds and flu as well as constipation-related hypertension and insomnia, as well as menopausal symptoms as well as sinusitis and back discomfort.

Chamomilla

In order for this remedy to be effective the patient will be prone to pain , and might have one cheek more red in comparison to the other. Patients may display an angry personality, be rude, irritable and sometimes violent. The conditions include asthma, diarrhoea and insomnia, menopausal and even withdrawal from drugs.

Hypericum-(St John's Wort)

It is also a common herbal remedy used to treat injuries or pain, but , in homoeopathic terms, it is typically used when there is a feeling of nerve pain nausea, nausea or stomach indigestion. Patients who respond well to it tend to be depressed and feel tired or in a state of forgetfulness, and their symptoms could be exacerbated by damp and cold. Hypericum can be helpful for headaches, depression diarrhoea, impotence and various types of injuries.

Nux vomica (Poison Nut)

While extremely poisonous in its natural form, it's safe to use as a homoeopathic cure. It can be beneficial to patients suffering from coughs, heartburn nausea, indigestion chills, vomiting, fevers, and so on. Patients can appear hostile, anxious, and aggressive or show a lack of reluctance. They might be insecure and frequently experience stress. Other issues include constipation, bladder infections diarrhoea and colds and Crohn's disease, nausea headaches, haemorrhoids kidney stones, insomnia, morning sickness, menopausal or hay fever.

Pulsatilla (Wind Flower)

Pulsatilla is a remedy for menstrual disturbances. Patients can experience psychological symptoms i.e. show signs of anxiety or moodiness and sensitive. Symptoms may become worse at night or in the night, and fluctuations in temperature can affect them as well. This remedy for homoeopathy is useful for asthma, arthritis and bronchitis. It can also help with stomach disorders, headaches fatigue, hay fever, morning sickness, headaches, etc.

Urtica urens (Stinging Nettle)

This remedy is useful for the treatment of joint sore throat, and skin that is blotchy This remedy is also used for gout, hives insect bites , arthritis such as rheumatoid, etc.

These are only a few examples of homeopathic remedies available and would need to be studied should you wish to pursue a course for a professional certificate in homeopathy.

If you're ready proceed then take a look at self-assessment Tasks and then review the new information you have learned.

Acupuncture

Another popular treatment to think about in addition to your naturopathic degree is acupuncture even though the training is lengthy. It requires a significant commitment to time, effort, and commitment to be certified, however it's an amazing therapy and, certainly, its benefits are vast.

Chinese medicine is deeply rooted in the past. Archaeologists have found acupuncture needles that date to when it was the Shang Dynasty. Within the Western the world we typically employ terms like Oriental medicine widely, however in reality, this doesn't even come close to determining the source of many of the traditional remedies and different countries have their own innovations in the field of healing research, both method and theory.

Over the past three thousand years, Oriental medicine has been capable of spreading throughout the globe. As a natural cure it's become commonplace. It is able to treat many illnesses, such as:

* Asthma

* The chronic fatigue syndrome

* Menopause symptoms

* Headaches

* Back and neck pain.

Reproductive health issues

* Insomnia

* Fibromyalgia

* Gastrointestinal problems

* Sports injuries etc.

You might be looking to learn more about acupuncture if have personal experience with sessions with acupuncture. Perhaps it helped you recover. It is possible that you are enthralled by an old-fashioned treatment that has shown results. Acupuncture is now a major part of the modern world It is recognized and accepted by conventional medicine and is widely regarded. It is a method of treatment that is a comprehensive method of diagnosis and treatment.

In taking care of patients, the goal is to ensure health by keeping life energy moving smoothly through channels known as meridians. Consider meridians as energy conduits that are in good condition. When they are opened and energy flow is free. If the conduit gets blocked, health issues appear. Within the body, emotional stress trauma, stress, injuries, and diseases all can disrupt the vital circulation of energy. As a result symptoms begin to show up.

The meridians

It isn't easy to visualize these meridian channels that extend all the way from your skin, linking all organs and tissues within the body. Though they're invisible but they are essential to know and be able recognize their location. In Oriental medical practices, meridians have been identified for a long time as essential to health since they carry energy, ensuring that your entire body gets well-nourished. While this is beneficial, it is important to note that blocked conduits may also carry diseases. This is the reason it is vital to be in a state of equilibrium in your life and to ensure that these meridians are free of any obstructions.

If you decide to learn about the practice of acupuncture, you'll come to realize that some patients may detect the area where the disruption of energy has taken place or, the issue could be manifesting in a different part of the body, and they are aware that something isn't right. Your job is to identify the source of the blockages and allow the energy to flow again so that it is able to flow again.

Acupuncture points

If you are able to translate the word acupuncture point into a literal translation the word acupuncture point means 'hole' and the position'.

These acupuncture points provide openings to meridians, so they can be accessed by internal organs and muscles. While it is not clear which method of healing the acupuncture method were first identified, the first documented in writing dates all the way to the 2nd century.

In the past, Acupuncture points were identified to meridians in accordance with the health benefits , and designated to describe their purpose. Acupuncture spots can be found on the major channels that run through the body upwards, downwards as well as sideways. like you see on the previous photo, it's a complicated system of meridians and acupuncture points , all of which need to be learned.

It is worth noting that a lot of the 361 points of meridian had been recognized by the end of the 3rd century. Other points were found in the ear that might also affect muscles and organs. Acupuncture points are typically located in the indentations of joints and muscles. If a spot is indicative of problems with health that are present, it is sensitive to pressure from the fingers. There's a lot of study required you can memorize the precise location of these points therefore, if you decide to specialize and incorporate this popular treatment into your repertoire, remember that it's an obligation in terms of time.

Acupuncture points are identified through proportional measurements of anatomical structures and this is simply a matter of equally measured measurements of every component will assist in finding the Acupuncture Point. It's not a precise method, but it can certainly aid. It can be done for everybody by taking your arm, breaking it down twelve units starting from their shoulder up to the elbow, and then allowing nine units to go from elbow up to the wrist. If you do this you will be within an approximate location of the appropriate acupuncture spot and then you can utilize your fingers to pinpoint the precise location.

Bio-electric flow

Scientists noticed an unpredictably occurring phenomenon during the study of acupuncture points. the electrical properties of the skin along these meridians as well as points of acupuncture were different from those areas with no acupuncture or meridian points. They discovered the fact that once an organ in the body is removed, the electrical power along the corresponding meridian could cease or disappear completely.

Research has revealed an energy system that interacts with the nervous system as well as the heart system. Certain of the changes that occur in the electrical currents of the skin have been proven to be linked directly to internal organs to the meridians. As with all developments, the latest advances in research will lead to more understanding and assessment.

Absolutely, human bodies comprises magnetic fields that are quantifiable. When magnets are placed directly on the acupuncture point and then they can be used to detect micro-currents within the nerves. This improves blood flow. The meridians' channels be responsive to the magnetic stimulus. To summarize that the body is comprised of many meridians, channels that connect the skin with organs, muscles, and nerves and acupuncture points provide pathways to access both inside and out of the body.

If you choose to pursue a course in the field of complementary health and, once you are qualified you need to be aware of the health issues that your clients face. Therefore, you'll look at the patient and try to determine what they look like. For instance are they energetic individuals who are full of energy, or are they thin in appearance or are they frail? The body type is observed along with facial tone, posture, and even the appearance on the skin.

The tongue is a diagnostic tool for the diagnosis of

The tongue is an vital aspect that is essential to Oriental diagnosis. It is connected to numerous of the meridian channels , and can also reflect the organs. You can observe the size, shape and even the color of your patient's tongue . Also, be aware of whether there is a an amorphous layer of tissue on top of the tongue. Also, check whether there are any bumps or fissures. The ideal tongue will appear pinkish and have the tongue having a thin white layer, but there must not be any bumps or marks on the sides.

Let's take a look at the possible issues:

If you notice the tongue has a thin, red tip it could mean that the individual is suffering from anxiety or emotional strains. of anxiety. A red tongue tip can indicate it is a sign that the emotions have been blocked, and can affect the way you sleep or your thoughts.

The tongue can be a helpful gauge of your health.

Also, you must check the patient's heart rate since, in Oriental medical practices The pulse is an indication of the health of the meridians as well as the organs that are associated to them. Along with the three pulse points on the wrists of each (the primary points to determine the pulse) every channel will have their own pulse points within the human body. In addition to checking the pulse as well as observing the tongue as well as the body in general and the body as a whole, it is important to go over medical history, take notes on their symptoms, and asking the patient what they prefer for cold or hot beverages and food preferences.

It may sound strange and may sound odd, but it is a way to construct an original and comprehensive overview of their health as well as of any illness. You must also be able to pay attention and to observe breath patterns in your patients, observing their speech patterns and also looking at the health of the acupuncture channels, acupuncture points as well as joints and identifying any soreness of meridians or acupuncture points since this could provide an unrivalled perspective on the health of the muscles and organ systems.

Many of your patients might not have had any experience with acupuncture, and might be a bit worried about the prospect of an aggressive treatment. They'll be reassured quickly because acupuncture does not cause pain. In the first place, acupuncture is safe when it is done by someone who is trained and skilled. The number of treatments that are performed is increasing every year, and there are few cases reported worldwide. However, acupuncture must be considered in some instances with extreme caution as per the following list:

* Women who are pregnant can be treated with acupuncture however it is recommended to stay clear of using points of acupuncture in the abdomen or in the lower back.

Acupuncture should never be administered to anyone who is using any recreational drug or are under the influence of alcohol.

* Acupuncture shouldn't be used for wounds that are open or if there are swellings that aren't diagnosed.

The needles, though quite long however, are very thin, and the treatment will not cause pain. Many people do not feel the needle is in and some are able to feel a tiny pressure. Feelings and sensations differ from individual to individual. As long as there isn't pain, this is normal.

Certain needles are placed in a shallow area just below the skin. Other needles might need to be located in the middle of a muscle or the joint. Some treatments require the needles to stay on the table for about 20 minutes. When this occurs, it's a ideal idea to play calming music so that the patient remains at ease and is able to relax. When you have an acupuncture session the body's system releases endorphins. These natural painkillers. Serotonin is released as well, which is the chemical that makes an person feel relaxed. The patient will notice it easier to release tension and perform normally. The circulation system of their body is enhanced.

Here are some fundamentals to be aware of during your exam:

Any edge that is serrated or teeth marks on the tongue can suggest digestive issues

* If there is a lot of heat inside the stomach or the lungs, breathing is likely to be sour.

* The tone of the skin and appearance of the face determine the health of your organs

The principal purpose of acupuncture is to keep life energy flowing effortlessly throughout your patient's body since when there is pain, energy becomes restricted and stagnant, and to relieve the pain, acupuncture needles are put along the meridian line to help move energy.

While the first acupuncture needles were made of stone, these days, the needles are ultra-fine, and are made from high-quality stainless steel, although some practitioners utilize electrical conductivity through zinc, gold, as well as copper needles. They are thin enough that when they penetrate the skin it isn't painful.

Re-usable needles or disposable ones are available.

While you are in training, you'll learn to use the needles through practicing on small pieces of fruit or foam in order you can learn the correct method. If the needles are placed swiftly and with care the patient will not feel any pain. There are various size and length of needles, and the choice you make will depend on the patient's physical and medical situation. It may be necessary to insert the needle, then remove it quickly, or keep the needle in place on the meridian lines for 20-30 minutes in order to clear any blocked energy.

After you have completed your training, you will be able to establish an intuitive approach to treating patients and be confident in diagnosing the problem areas and repairing. If you're prepared to complete the self-assessment, start now. If you are unable to answer one of the questions, make sure to go back to the course and read the material again.

Self-Assessment Tasks

Task:

What are the acupuncture needles usually constructed from?

Task:

Why is the importance of the tongue so great?

Task:

What does the word "acupuncture point" mean?

Task:

How do I define meridians?

Be aware that these self-assessment exercises are designed to test your understanding of the material in each module. So, don't send them in for review to KEW Training Academy.

Herbalism

If you're curious about herbal medicine, be aware that it's an interesting yet complex field that takes dedication and patience. It can be a key component to your naturopathy set, and allow you to assist lot of people, as it has a loyal following and, in recent years, has entered the mainstream of healing.

When you study herbs , you can access the natural pharmacy of nature and learn how to create skincare solutions including natural baths, tonics, herbal bouquets, poultices and tisanes. It is important to know the background of health benefits from herbs and how it's evolved through the ages. Understanding how to grow and maintain your herbs is a crucial aspect particularly if you intend to cultivate your own herbs to use in your own practice.

There are:

* Astringent herbs

* Antispasmodic herbs

* Expectant herbs

* Herbs that are purgative

* Diuretic herbs

Learn about cleansing regimens and how to gain an intuitive understanding of the health concerns of your client.

So, what exactly is herbal medicine?

If you go through the dictionary, you will find that there are two definitions for herb.

"A plant that produces seeds but doesn't develop long-lasting woody tissue, but dies in the middle to the growth season."

The second, generally based definition often employed:

"A plant or part of a plant appreciated because of its medicinal or savory or aromatic properties."

This implies that a plant or plant component could be utilized .....so for example, the tree's bark the leaf, a root an acorn, a flower or indeed any other plant part in the event that it is being used to enhance the aroma of the plant to enhance savoury dishes or to treat ailments.

* Savoury is a term used to describe herbs that can be used to flavor food.

* Aromatic is a term used to describe the plants or herbs which are utilized in perfumes or scents, etc.

*Medicinal is the term used to describe the plants used in treating and preventing diseases.

Herbalists prefer using the whole herb , and believe that it will result in less side effects as opposed to when pharmaceutical companies attempt to isolate chemicals in order to make an undiluted concentrate that could be used in conventional medicine. Therefore herbal medicine refers to the use of plant's seeds or flowers, roots, berries or leaves used to treat ailments. It's also known as phytomedicine or botanical medicine.

The use of herbal medicine is a long tradition of use outside the realm of conventional medicine, however due to advancements in clinical research , which demonstrate the effectiveness of herbal medicine in the treatment and prevention of diseases and disease - it is becoming more popular. Each herb is composed of naturally occurring chemical compounds and even in the present day and age, it's safe to say that the functions of several of these chemicals aren't fully understood. Some chemicals are synergistic and others alter the effects of other chemicals. The fact is that when you combine the entire herb, you will get greater outcomes. Nature seems to know best.

There is a chance that you have heard of the term "active," it refers to what is called the active ingredient in the herb. As an instance, when we look at St John's wort, the active ingredients are hyperforin and hypericin. This can be helpful for testing or standardisation however, the active ingredients aren't the only beneficial ingredient which can be found in the herb. So pharmaceutical companies frequently make this error and get a medicine that do not provide better results over the natural herb.

The background

The antiquated Chinese and Egyptians have reported the medicinal properties of plants back to 3000 BC. Other cultures, such as Native Americans have also long utilized herbs in their own healing rituals. Studies show that similar or identical plants are used predominantly for the same purpose across the globe. This suggests that there is a certain amount of accuracy in the use of herbal medicine.

Recent research suggests that 80percent of the population around the world use herbal remedies for certain aspect of health.

When chemical analysis was first made accessible in the 19th century scientists were able take and alter the active components of plants and started to formulate their own versions of these chemicals and, consequently, the health emphasis shifted towards pharmaceuticals. Since the majority of these compounds utilized only active ingredients and did not provide any results in terms of health benefits. In recent times, many are returning to the belief of natural wellness as superior to relying on prescription drugs which can have a number of side effects.

What are the effects of herbs?

The problem with scientists extracting an active ingredient and altering it is that the whole herb has several ingredients working in tandem to provide a beneficial impact. However, in addition it is possible that there are additional aspects to take into consideration:

* The climate

* Soil quality

* Harvesting time

* Processing

What are the uses of herbs?

Herbal supplements have seen a dramatic increase in the last few decades. The supplements are classified under the category of supplements, and therefore, unlike prescription drugs , they can be sold without testing to make sure they are safe and of course and effective.

The most frequently taken herbal supplements are:

* Echinacea (Echinacea purpurea)

* Garlic (Allium sativum)

* Ginseng (Panax ginseng, Asian ginseng)

* Goldenseal (Hydrastis Canadensis)

* Chamomile (Matricaria recutita)

* Feverfew (Tanacetum parthenium)

* Evening Primrose (Oenothera biennis)

* Milk Thistle (Silybum marianum)

Herbal medicine is a great option to treat a variety of health issues such as:

* Allergies

* Asthma

* Premenstrual syndrome

* Fibromyalgia

* Rheumatoid arthritis

* Menopausal symptoms

* Chronic fatigue

* Cancer

* Irritable bowel syndrome

It is always recommended for anyone considering taking herbal remedies for the first time , to consult a licensed herbalist due to the possibility that prescription drugs might interfere with the herbal remedies , and that could cause a worsening of any medical condition. It is important to take this into consideration when you are beginning your natural medicine practice. It is important to check any medication a patient might be taking.

Some common herbs:

Ginkgo (Ginkgo biloba)

It is a well-known herb that can be used to combat the effects of the symptoms of dementia, poor circulation and also to improve memory. Research has shown that blood circulation improves when you take this herb because it dilates blood vessels, and ginkgo decreases the adherence that blood platelets have. It is important to take care of patients who are taking blood thinners, as would anyone who has an epilepsy history or those who have fertility problems.

Saw palmetto (Serenoa repens)

It is the herb that is that is used by millions of men to treat benign prostate hyperplasia (BPH)

that's a benign, non-cancerous growth of the prostate gland. It is a non-cancerous enlargement of the. Studies have shown that this herb can be effective in alleviating symptoms such as issues with urination as well as who need to urinate at night.

St. John's wort (Hypericum perforatum)

It is a widely-known herb frequently used to treat depression due to its effects. Studies have shown that it is a good choice successfully for people who suffer from moderate to mild depression, and can cause lower side effects than many prescribed medicines. When taking any prescribed medication be sure to check the fact that St John's wort doesn't interfere with the medication and should not be taken in conjunction with prescribed antidepressants.

Valerian (Valeriana officinalis)

Valerian is a very well-known herbal remedy used to reduce sleep disorders. Valerian is less prone to negative effects than prescribed sleeping tablets, as they typically induce morning sleepiness. It is able to interact with prescription medication, therefore care should be taken.

Echinacea products (from Echinacea purpurea)

Echinacea is a popular herb remedy that aids in improving natural immunity within the body. It is among the most widely used herbal treatments. It is not recommended to take for long periods of time and can be a drug interaction, which means it could not be suitable for everyone, particularly people suffering from autoimmune disorders.

If used properly the herbal products can aid in treating a range of health issues and surely have fewer adverse side consequences than prescribed medications. There are many reasons to be concerned. be when you purchase herbal products on online or on the Internet or purchase them from an unidentified source, as the product is often not properly labeled, and they could contain ingredients or substances which are not mentioned as ingredients on the labels. Furthermore, some herbs may be harmful in the event that they are not handled correctly.

Here are a few examples of how herbs may cause issues:

We've stated before the fact that St John's wort is an effective treatment for people who are feeling down or suffers from mild depression. However, this herb may make the skin have increased sensitivity to sun's ultraviolet rays. It can cause nausea, stomach upset and even allergic reactions. While it is beneficial, as we've already stated it should not be taken in conjunction with any prescription antidepressant medications. Also , there are contraindications when it is taken in conjunction with birth medications for asthma control, birth control pills as well as blood thinners.

For certain people, Valerian could be stimulating instead of relaxing. Evening Primrose can increase the amount of seizures suffered by patients who already suffer from seizures, and feverfew. ginger and ginkgo can increase the chance of bleeding.

This highlights the necessity for licensed herbalists who are able to guide clients in a safe manner to ensure there are no contraindications and are experienced

Herbs are available in variety of forms that include:

* Teas

* Tinctures

* Dry extracts

* Syrups

* Liquid extracts

* Oils

It is simple to make teas with dried herbs. The herb can be prepared by soaking it for some minutes in boiling or hot water before straining the liquid. The oils come from plants and are great for use in creams, ointments, or ointments. They can also as massage rubs. Tinctures are created when active herb ingredients are dissolving in an alcohol-based solution (often alcohol) and usually have a 1.5 and 1.10 concentration. In simple terms, it is the case when one component from the plant is prepared by mixing 5-10 parts (weight) of liquid. Liquid extracts can be prepared similar manner, however they are much more concentrated than the tinctures, and typically 1.1 concentration. Tablets, capsules, or even lozenges are made by the process of dry extracts and the most concentrated versions are typically: 2.1 -8.1.

While the majority of herbal remedies bought are safe, it's important to note that there is no official authority that oversees the production or identification of herbal products. This means that there is no method to guarantee the quantity of herbs contained in the bottle, which could result in incorrect dosages being consumed. Certain herbal products however that are standardized and thus assures the amount of active ingredients in the herb.

Many doctors and professionals utilize herbal remedies in their personal treatments, including:

* Herbalists

* Physicians

* Medical doctors

* Chinese medicine practitioners

* Naturopathic doctors

As you'll have learned by studying this course an naturopath believes that the body needs equilibrium to be healthy and that natural remedies help to achieve this. This is why naturopathy training, typically takes place over four years incorporates courses in medical sciences such as pathology for instance as well as clinical training in nutrition, lifestyle counseling homoeopathy, or herbal medicine. It is possible to select the topics that are studied, and herbal medicine is certainly well-known and intriguing in its many forms.

If you think about the fact that the first recorded record for herbal medicines was made more than five thousand years ago in the the ancient Mesopotamia and there are no doubts that the use of herbal medicine will continue to be in use. Through the years people have relied on plants to nourish themselves and have discovered through experimentation and trial that some can be beneficial for nutrition. However, certain plants are poisonous , while some may cause hallucinogenic effects as well as plants that aid in healing or ease discomfort. Every generation of herbalists has developed and refined their knowledge of the herbs.

The origins of Chinese medicine that has been heavily affected by herbal medicine has a history of around 500 years. In addition, the Chinese medicinal herbal text called Pen Tsao contains details of more than 300 plants. In India sacred writings are found to the second century. Their medical system is called"the Ayurveda as well as the listing of plants that are used for treatment is vast. Ayurvedic herbalism is still in use in the present day.

It's likely to be true to say that Greeks and Romans have a great deal of their knowledge of herbs from the early civilisations. Hippocrates the Greek doctor, whom we often refer to as the "father of modern medicine was actually an herbalist.

The majority of herbs were utilized throughout the world throughout in the Middle Ages in Europe and America and during this time of time, the understanding of herbal remedies grew significantly as monks analyzed the benefits of medicinal plants they cultivated.

Herbalism Today

In the past herbalism has always been connected to superstition and magic however, the practice of the present is quite different due to the fact that the use of scientific methods is used to determine the curative properties of these traditional plants. In various different ways, this research has revived the curiosity in herbalism, and allowed modern society to recognize the herbs that are efficient and safe to utilize. Furthermore that we can utilize herbs that aren't only available in our area, but also get herbs from all over the globe.

A lot of herbs have been harvested too much but this includes golden seal root as well as wild American Ginseng, so there's an element of concern. However, less prosperous nations could turn away from the use of rain forests to harvest agricultural crops and instead pick their own local plants.

It is common to hear herbs being used as an alternative treatment, however in reality, herbal remedies have been in use for a longer time than Western medications. If you think about the fact that the majority of the drugs used today are only around for some time or just a few years, you can understand why people put more confidence in herbal remedies. .Some herbal remedies are able to be utilized at home, but the majority of herbs can provide positive health benefits every day basis.

Ginger (Zingiber officinale)

Ginger is believed to improve digestion and increase appetite. Small amounts from ginger are also found to be effective for morning sickness.

Marshmallow (Althaea officinalis)

Marshmallow root has been utilized to treat a variety of illnesses, including lung and bronchial issues like coughs, mucus, and Emphysema. However, it has also been utilized to remove kidney stones as well as to treat ulcers.

Slippery Elm (Ulmus fulva)

Slippery elm has been traditionally used to treat sore throats and when respiratory dryness tract is observed. It is also utilized to treat sores and open wounds, and to treat diarrhoea and hemorrhoids.

Studying herbal treatments is an interesting and intricate one, as there's a lot to know. This guide will provide you with an insight into the possibility of you include medical herbalism in your list of credentials. If you're happy with the knowledge contained in this module and you are ready to begin the self-study assessment take them. If you are having difficulty solving any of the questions, make sure to go carefully through the content of this course before going on.

Chapter 8: Self-Study Assessment

Task:

The benefits of ginger are listed below.

Task:

Three of the most loved supplements

Task:

The following list of 3 conditions can be treated with herbs

Note that these self-assessment exercises will ensure that you understand of the content in each module. So, do not submit them to KEW Training Academy for review. KEW Training Academy.

Nutrition

Learning more about the field of nutrition could be very beneficial to your profession as a naturopath . It also, naturally, it will benefit many of your clients since you'll be able to help them navigate the complex world of nutrition.

The world is changing constantly and we're being offered food products that may not be what we would expect. The labels can be misleading, and even the advertised 'healthy food might not be as healthy as they appear. Knowing why is the best way to help your clients meet their nutritional requirements.

The society we live in today is quite different from the previous years in that fewer people have the time to focus on the essentials of living. Food is among those things that are usually not thought of in the sense of importance. it's simple to buy prepared meals or quickly warm something in the microwave. It's easy to see how this kind of living becomes routine. In actual fact there are only a few people who can claim that they've never eaten processed or pre-packaged food before.

The world of today is controlled through the influence of media. We are bombarded by advertisements all day. Even when we're careful about what we eat, a portion of the information is still making into our minds and is stored within the subconscious mind. If you go through the aisles of a grocery store and buy a new item most of the time, you're reacting to advertisements that have been repeated every day. It is possible that we are not conscious of it, but it's an unconscious process since we are exposed to the same images repeatedly and the message that is behind them is in our heads.

You are probably aware of this, however the power of marketing is extremely strong, but often not accurate. Your customers will have similar experiences, and a lot will be afflicted with negative feelings about food.

Although you'll care about the health of your customers but the issue is that food producers do not. There's an abundance of psychological factors that affect the way a product is advertised to the general public. It is often the case that ingredients such as sugar and salt are disguised with different terms. Almost all processed items contain sugar and salt. Other ingredients include the addition of colourings as well as E number. In essence, people do not know what food they are eating.

As per the law in many countries it is required to provide an indication of these ingredients on the package, but since very few people know what they are this warning is often ignored. Food that is processed or packaged will contain preservatives as well. If a food item has to go through a number of steps in a manufacturing facility before it is put on the shelves of the supermarket, then it's no longer a real food.

Food producers spotted a demand and took advantage of it in the form of convenience food items. There are many people who live a hectic life eating in the rush or snack, and get tired at the time they are done. Many times, they are too exhausted to cook from scratch once they return home, they make themselves promise to eat to eat a nutritious meal the next day and the pattern continues. A lot of people nowadays live a hectic life and feed their families with low quality food items that have little nutritional value. Often, include harmful ingredients.

You can see the importance of understand nutrition.

It is essential to know what is going on inside our bodies in order to assist our fellow humans and ourselves. Having a the concept of nutrition as an additional certification to your naturopathy degree could prove very beneficial.

To be able to assist clients, you must be able to at least have a basic understanding of not only the reason the issue is there, but also be able to correct it. Also, we must be aware of what the body requires in order for optimal functioning. This module will help you understand everything.

What exactly does nutrition mean?

The essence of nutrition is how the body absorbs minerals and vitamins and converts it into use by the body. The nutritional value is the measure of the amount of nutritional benefit that can be obtained from a particular food item and to provide us with more understanding that it is important to know what we really require to live healthy, active life.

It is essential to eat all nutrients in a consistent manner, which includes:

* Fats

Minerals

* Carbohydrates

* Proteins etc.

Minerals and vitamins are required to ensure that we have the health of our bones and skin, and, more importantly, to ensure that all bodily functions function. It is important to note that water is essential every day and , although it's not an essential nutrient, it helps the body in different ways. It is possible to live without food for a while but then quickly go to a decline with no water.

It is important since it aids digestion and keeps the body at a healthy temperature, and also helps eliminate waste materials out of the body as well. A majority of our water is derived from eating food that is composed of vegetables and fruits however drinking fresh water is also a must. If you are thirsty, you're in the process of becoming dehydrated, as your body begging for water to replenish what it has lost.

It's crucial to remember the fact that whenever you're feeling thirsty your body is requesting water, not some calories sugar-laden, chemically enhanced, fizzy drink.

Let's take a closer look at the various elements our bodies require.

Vitamins

Vitamins are an organic compound that is an essential nutrient which is available through a variety of food items.

Vitamins can be listed in two different sections.

Fat soluble vitamins

These vitamins can live in the fat cells of our bodies for weeks , or in some instances, even months. The body keeps fat-soluble vitamins in reserve in case of emergency.

Water-soluble vitamins

They are not stored in the body in any way, and if you absorb more than required, you will eliminate them via urine. Vitamins that are water-soluble need to be replaced regularly.

Here's a list with the most important vitamins.

Water-soluble

Vitamin B1... found in seeds and nuts, as well as whole grain cereals

Vitamin B2... It is present in whole grains the liver, nuts, seeds

Vitamin B3... It is found in fish, meat, poultry, and whole grains

Vitamin B5... It is found in chicken, meat and then whole grain

Vitamin B6... You will find this in fortified cereals as well as soya-based products.

Vitamin B6... It is found in meats and fruits

Vitamin B9... The primary source of vitamin B9 is in leafy green vegetables.

Vitamin B12... In the meat, poultry, fish and dairy products

Vitamin C... Most commonly found in citrus juices and fruits, and as well as in yellow, red and green peppers.

Fat-soluble

Vitamins A... are found in orange-coloured fruit and vegetables. It is also found within dark and leafy greens such as Kale

Vitamin D... It is found in fortified dairy products and milk such as cereals, as well as in sunshine

Vitamin E... It is also is found in cereals with fortification, leavesy vegetables and greens, nuts and seeds

Vitamin K... This vitamin is present on dark leafy vegetables , beetroots, turnips and beetroots.

It is essential to know the function of each vitamin in your body.

Vitamin B1 is essential to assist in metabolism and energy, it is also used to improve nerve function.

Vitamin B 2, also known as vitamin B2, is utilized in energy metabolism, but also helps with the skin and vision.

Vitamin B 3 is utilized in the metabolism of energy, however it is also a vital function for the nervous system as well as in the digestive system as well It also aids in helping to keep skin health in check.

Vitamin B6 assists in the metabolism of proteins and aids in the production of red blood cells.

Vitamin B12 is essential for the nervous system and brain as well as helping to create new cells.

Vitamin C aids in protein metabolism and helps to boost with the defense system. It also assists in the absorption of iron.

Vitamin A has numerous uses and is primarily required for vision , but also to maintain healthy mucous membranes, skin and is used to boost bone growth and immune.

Vitamin D is essential for calcium absorption.

Vitamin E helps defend cells and is beneficial for the skin.

Vitamin K is required to ensure the proper blood clotting process.

A balanced diet must provide the person with all the necessary minerals and vitamins, but when it is not possible to do so it is possible to require supplements. People who are on restricted diets i.e. vegetarians might require supplements.

Let's look at fats, which are another important ingredient in our health. There are two primary types of fats: transfats, and saturated fats.

Trans-fats are created through processing and are utilized for fast food outlets since processing methods also increase the shelf-life of the food item but trans-fats are by far the most detrimental type for your body since they cause bad cholesterol and increase the levels of heart disease and obesity in any society that utilizes these types of fats. There are trans-fats present in the majority of pastries, biscuits and cakes. In most cases, the term trans-fats is not mentioned, but look at the labels and you could be able to see an oil that has been hydrogenated. This is another example of how food companies try to deceive us.

Saturated fats are commonly found in red meats and dairy products. They also increase blood cholesterol levels and raise the risk of developing heart disease, though it is believed that a small amount of saturated fats can be beneficial in all diets. They are referred to as saturated fats since they change into solid when heated to room temperature.

Mono-saturated fat is believed to provide some benefits to the diabetic diet since they can boost blood cholesterol levels. they are typically found in oils.

Polyunsaturated fats are typically found in plant-based food items and are considered to be a great fat to add to your diet.

Omega-3 fatty acids can be found in many plant-based foods , but they are most commonly found in fish that are fatty. Research has shown that Omega fats were beneficial for heart health, however, there's still plenty of research needed in this field.

Cholesterol is often criticized and there are many misconceptions about this substance produced by our body naturally , and is crucial. We are constantly told about cholesterol, both good and bad, and, in fact, there are two types of. Good cholesterol is responsible for the creation of certain hormones that repair cells in the body. However, excessive levels of cholesterol generally means that there is excessive amounts in the form of bad cholesterol, and it could block arteries and trigger numerous cardio-related issues. A large portion of cholesterol comes from our diets and is found in dairy products, meat and eggs.

When discussing lifestyles and diets with your client, it's essential to include minerals as they are often overlooked since we only require small amounts of these. A typical diet should contain all the essential minerals but it's worth checking. It is likely that if someone has in a way that is influenced by media and eats a lot of processed food items in their diet, they may be missing vital minerals, putting themselves at risk of health issues.

On packaging for food items the salt ingredient is usually concealed but you can see sodium listed. It's true that salt is a component but as an elemental mineral sodium is crucial. It's only when you consume it in large quantities that it can become an issue. It can raise blood pressure. It can also alter the taste senses. It is essential to maintain fluid balance and plays an important role in the contraction of muscles. Thus, a small amount sodium is vital, however it is not necessary to add it into our diets because it's readily found in milk, sauces breads, vegetable, and some raw meats.

Potassium is a lot like sodium in that it does the same job as sodium does in that it assists in the balance of fluids as well as nerve transmission and muscle contraction. It is present in milk, meats as well as in fruits and vegetables and also in grains.

The majority of people are familiar with calcium, and understand that it's essential to dental health and bones however, it also assists muscles stretch and relax. Additionally, assists in other areas too, including the regulation of blood pressure and the immune system, and nerve function. It's readily accessible in milk products and in canned fish that have bones like sardines. It's found in fortified tofu as well as various dark green leafy veggies.

Phosphorus is vital for healthy teeth and bones too. It can be found in every cell, and plays a crucial function in maintaining the balance of acid. It is simple to locate since it is present in a variety of foods that are likely to be part of the typical diet, such as fish, meat eggs, poultry and milk. It is also found in certain processed food items.

Magnesium can be found in bones. It is a key element in the production of protein. It is also involved with other minerals to aid in the growth of our immune system. In addition, it isn't difficult to find through a healthy diet since it can be found in seeds, nuts and leafy green vegetables. seafood as well as chocolate, artichokes, as well as in drinking water that is hard to drink.

Sulphur is a small amount required since it is essential to form protein molecules. It can be found in poultry, meat eggs, fish, milk , and even nuts.

A lot minerals are omitted or deemed unimportant, but they all are essential in tiny amounts, therefore it is simple to get enough mineral levels if you're eating a balanced and healthy diet. There are additional minerals that are also needed by the body, but in lesser amounts. These are referred to as trace minerals.

It is an element that can be traced. it is the red blood cells, which is vital for transporting oxygen throughout the body. Therefore, it is an important part of the metabolism of energy. A majority of people obtain sufficient iron from red meats such as fish, poultry as well as shellfish, eggs, dried fruits and egg yolks along with dark, leafy vegetables.

Zinc is also a vitally crucial role in the body because it's used in creating proteins and genetic material. It aids in gaining the ability to detect taste. It is crucial to produce the sperm and plays other functions in the health of our immune system as well as aiding in healing wounds. It is found in fish, meats as well as whole grains, poultry and in vegetables.

Iodine is present in the thyroid hormone . It aids in regulating growth of the metabolism. You can find it in seafood or in foods made from soil that is rich but bread and dairy products too contain Iodine.

Selenium is an antioxidant. It is present in fish, meats and even grains.

Copper aids the metabolism of iron. It is available in seeds and nuts, as well as whole grains as well as drinking water.

Chromium - This trace mineral is in close contact with insulin, and is essential for the control in blood sugar levels. It is present in many unprocessed foods.

Fluoride is an elemental trace mineral that frequently gets a bad rap, but remains essential, even in small amounts. It aids in the development of bones and teeth . It also helps prevent tooth decay. Certain drinking water supplies contain fluoride, and it's also present in fish.

Carbohydrates

This is where the energy required by the body is derived. However, there is a huge difference between a processed and a complete carb. Processed carbohydrates , which are that are found in pastries, cakes and other processed foods trigger huge spikes in the levels of glucose in blood. In the event of this, the body experiences a surge of energy. This can be followed up by a sluggish response. Carbohydrates derived from whole food sources release energy gradually throughout the day or, at the very least, over several hours.

The body requires proteins to function properly and proteins break down within the body into different amino acids, and utilized in a variety of ways. One of the major benefits of protein is in the transport of nutrients to the right areas of the body.

It may appear like a lot of information, but this is only a small portion of the vital nutritional knowledge that you can acquire by doing this study as an additional component to your naturopathy certification.

If you take the advice listed in this article, you'll be able to see how crucial it is to comprehend the importance of foods do to the body , and also the challenges faced by people who don't follow a healthy diet...fatigue or weight gain digestive issues etc.

It is essential to establish an improved relationship with food, and also recognize the power of marketing companies that could mislead us when we're not cautious. If you examine this topic, you can easily see an interplay between the way food producers market their products that are of no nutritional value to us and how nutritionally inadequate diets can lead to health issues.

Nutrition is an intriguing and complex topic, therefore, by thoroughly studying nutrition you'll be able assist others in making better choices regarding their diets and begin the healing process by ensuring that their bodies are stocked with the essential nutrients they require. Learning about nutrition can be an excellent addition to any profession.

Self-Assessment Test

Task:

What is the primary distinction between wholefood and processed carbohydrates?

Task:

Is there a mineral called a trace?

Task:

Choose one fat that are actually beneficial to you.

Task:

Name 4 minerals present in dairy or meat products.

Note the self-assessment assignments are designed to test your understanding of the content in each module. Therefore, don't send them in for review to KEW Training Academy.

Introduction to Iridology

There are numerous diagnostic techniques that are used in natural medicine however Iridology is a great one and should you decide to add it to your certification in Naturopathy it will allow you to gain a better knowledge of the client's present health condition.

It is possible to gain valuable information on the health of organs and tissues in the body by studying eyes. While conventional tests can only show that an organ or an area of the body has been damaged Iridology can reveal any organ that is suffering from stress , which can trigger changes.

Iridology isn't a new concept It has been around since the seventeenth Century and throughout the years there has been a lot of study conducted into the iris markings and potential significance. One of the first researchers was Dr. Ignatz von Peczely the Hungarian Doctor. In his youth, he injured the wing of an owl. It broke it. He noticed the appearance of a black mark in the eye of the owl, which in time, began to change as healing began.

He completed his medical studies in The Vienna Medical College in 1867 and was able to observe eye movements of his patients prior to or after surgery. He wrote down all his observations, and created his Iris Chart was created in 1880.

In the early 1860s In the 1860s, a Swedish boy named Nils Liljequist was ill after the vaccination process. After receiving doses of quinine and iodine and quinine, he noticed changes happening to his eyes that were blue. He could spot spots of drug in the form they appear. In the wake of this, he wrote the results of his experience, stating the possibility that quinine or iodine change the color of the iris.

In the US Medical research started by the Dr. Henry Edward Lane and his pupil Dr. Henry Lindlahr. The Dr. Lane did much of his autopsy and surgical connections in Iridology within Illinois. After conducting research on thousands of patients the author published his book Iridology: The Diagnosis of the Eye in 1904.

Dr. J Haskel Kritzer also recorded his findings that were gathered from a long period of research in his book entitled "Iridiagnosis." This work later prompted Bernard Jensen to continue the research by releasing an updated Iris Chart - along with Dr. John R Arnold, who was the creator of the "World Iridology Foundation'. The doctor. Arnold who changed the name from "iridiagnosis" to the term 'iris analysis'. This accurately conveys the fact that Iridology is a way to study 'health issues instead of being able to diagnose specific illnesses.

Iridology is a unique treatment, but it is well-regarded. It lets you learn much more about the health of people around you by the examination of their eyes, instead of through the art of communicating. In an Iridology test it is the Iris, the sclera and pupil, as well as the pupil border, and collaret are inspected.

The optic nerve that is located in the eyes is accountable for transmitting all information about the visual that is received with the brain. The brain relays information back towards the eye. The Iris is like fingerprints and, with the same thought in place, it is only natural that many security organizations use biotechnology and identification using the eyes to identify themselves as security tools.

Absolutely the patterns and colours of the fibres in them reveal physical and emotional issues for up to three generations behind. Iridology is also utilized to determine the strength of the body. It aids in the evaluation of personality traits too. These traits are influenced by subconscious and conscious patterns of thought. If you're considering the study of Iridology It is important to know that it's not meant to be used for treatment, rather it is an instrument for diagnosing. However, it can be utilized as a preventative method to prevent any disease before it becomes more severe and even life-threatening. It is not painful and non-evasive and may reveal a lot of information about the person:

• Genetic weakness and strength

* Identifies the organs that might be troublesome

* Reveals strength of the constitution

* Identifies the type of personality

* Identifies the function of the nervous system.

It cannot be revealed:

* The real disease

* The condition of the tissue function

• The existence of an infection.

Exercise, diet, or lifestyle changes

Constitution

Constitution is the result of the mix of strengths and weaknesses you inherit through your grandparents. Therefore, this part of iridology is determined by genetics. Your parents will have specific traits, however it is important to remember that your spiritual, emotional and physical abilities develop as you get into adulthood. These abilities also evolve through the experiences in your the course of life.

Understanding the constitution of your body, it enables you identify weak points which may be present but can also, in a positive way helps you support and enhance your energy force. Therefore, Iridology recognizes three types of constitutions:

Strong Constitution

People with a strong constitution typically tend to take care of themselves less physically since they are convinced that they won't experience any negative consequences in the form of. They do not even think about their health at all as they believe they are not required to consider it. People with a strong constitution have a tendency to recover faster from health issues, and tend to be less tolerant to those who may take longer to heal from ailments.

Medium constitution

Individuals with moderate constitutions will typically suffer from more weakening in their bodies. To be healthy, they must tend to themselves and don't forget to the opportunity to treat their bodies, knowing that they can't be allowed to do it. In the end, they are more conscious of what they eat, the environment they consume, where they live , and the environment where they work, etc. They are also more sensitive and demonstrate compassion towards those sick. They usually are drawn to jobs that involve taking care of other people.

A weak constitution

More attention is required for those with weaker constitution. They need to work more hard to heal and stay healthy.

Personality kinds

We've previously mentioned that Iridology is a way to identify personality types . This is covered under the category of behavioural Iridology. Everyone has different methods of communicating our needs. the process of learning and behavioural iridology could help an individual to become more conscious and aware of their feelings and this could be helpful in preventing physical ailments or ailments.

Most introverts are analytical in their approach. They are physically kinaesthetic. They often have an impressive constitution. Extroverts, on the other hand, tend to be more emotionally and fast-paced, but they typically be weaker in their constitution and needs to be nurtured.

Base colors

In iridology, there are 3 authentic base colours that are recognized. Each color is associated with specific characteristics.

Blue eyes:

Hair with blonde or fair complexions typically have blue eyes. Some health markers include

• Allergies, asthma and allergies.

* Insufficiency of your upper respiratory system

* High acidity from high pressure

* The arteries become more hardened as we the ages

* Inflammatory conditions such as arthritis.

* The throat, ear and nose issues in the early years of childhood.

* Skin conditions such as eczema and eczema.

* Brown eyes

People with dark hair and olive skin tones typically have brown eyes. Some health concerns include:

* Liver congestion

* Poor circulation

* Haemorrhoids and thrombosis

* Anaemia

* Irritability that increases with age

* Digestive disorders

* Hormonal disturbances

Eyes mixed

The blue-brown mixed eye health indicators comprise:

* Food sensitivities

* Gallstones

* Glandular conditions

* Constipation

* Flatulence

* Gallbladder disorders

* Sleep pattern disturbances

* Headaches

If you choose to be certified in Iridology in the future, you'll often be able to see colour patterns based on the exact location of the iris. You will then compare them with Iridology charts. Here's an illustration:

White

White is usually the sign of early stage inflammation at the beginning of. When there's a broad splash of white on blue eyes, one should look for a diagnosis of arthritis, gout or high concentrations of acid. The appearance of this will be an orange or grade tint in people with brown eyes. If there are white fibers in an organ that indicates an overactive thyroid gland, and any white spotted within the region in the thyroid gland will be a sign of hypothyroidism.

Yellow

If the area is yellow, this indicates that kidneys aren't functioning properly. Spots of yellow in particular organs could indicate acute inflammation in that organ.

Orange

If the color orange is evident it indicates that any health issue is advancing towards becoming long-term. Pancreatic and blood tests might be necessary. If there is a discoloration of orange in relation to an organ, it could indicate an inactivity.

Brown

Brown color can indicate an intoxic or weak liver. This is usually in a long-term stage, so detoxification is required. If there is a brown discoloration within the organ this could indicate the presence of pathological changes.

Black

If there is a black discoloration that indicates necrosis or degeneration of an part.

This concludes the short intro to Iridology and, if you're prepared, you can move on to the self-assessment questions. Make sure you take your time when completing these tasks to ensure that you have a complete understanding of the content in this module.

Self-Assessment Task

Task:

What does constitution mean?

Task:

What does white mean to the eyes?

Task:

What do yellow flecks symbolize to the eyes?

Task:

What are the three base colours of your eyes?

Task:

Can Iridology be used to treat health problems?

Be aware the self-assessment assignments are designed to test your understanding of the content in each module. So, do not submit them to KEW Training Academy for review. KEW Training Academy.

Flower Remedies

Flowers are used in a variety of ways and most well-known is the one developed by Dr. Edward Bach who concluded that when patients experience emotional problems, the correct flower essence could help aid in healing the issue. Bach was a physician but also had an fascination with homeopathy. He stepped away from his traditional medical practice to learn the true essence of flowers.

When Bach began treating patients with flowers, he began to realize what he needed to watch out for and treat. These were the signs not just from the body but also the heart and mind.

Bach passed away in 1936, however he left behind a legacy. Nowadays, increasing numbers of individuals are moving away treatments and are seeking alternative therapies that are holistic. Bach believed that how people perceive and experience their thoughts is connected with the effects they have on their physical body . This is taken into consideration by doctors of the present.

Bach was also influenced by Dr. Samuel Hahnemann who was the creator of what we now know as homoeopathy and as a result, he began to group his patients into types and then look at how to treat them. He believed that people were supposed to exist in harmony with nature and that nature could cure illness. He believed that people had turned away from respecting and caring for nature and it was because of this that people were more prone to illness. At the time, many doctors and the general public were disbelieving about all that he said, they could not believe that a flower essence would be strong enough to be able to deal with illness of any sort.

Initially Bach collected dew drops on the flowers as he believed that the essence of the flower (energy) would pass into the water but then realised that this was not sufficient so he began to mix these dew drops with brandy and then diluted it yet further before giving to his patients. He found that this was still insufficient so he began to suspend the flowers in spring water and allow the energy from the sun to pass through them, he believed that as a result, the water would then be energised with the power of the flower essence.

Bach was convinced that the essence was akin to a vibrational imprint left behind by the flower and as each flower held different vibrations, it would change to the nature of that illness. Bach could see that the flower essences could increase energy levels and change negative mental states to a more positive one. He realised that even if a patient took the wrong flower remedy, there would be no negative side effects and so these remedies were safe.

There are 38 actual flower remedies and they are as follows:

- Agrimoney
- Aspen
- Beech
- Centaury
- Cerato
- cherry plum
- Chestnut Bud
- Chicory
- Clematis
- Crabapple
- Elm
- Gentian
- Gorse
- Heather
- Holly
- Honeysuckle

- Hornbeam
- Impatiens
- Larch
- Mimulus
- Mustard
- Oak
- Olive
- Pine
- Red Chestnut
- Rock rose
- Rock water
- Scleranthus
- Star of Bethlehem
- Sweet chestnut
- Vervain
- Vine
- Walnuts

- Water violet
- White chestnuts
- White Oat
- Wild Rose
- Willow

And…Rescue Remedy.

Conclusion

Naturopathy can enhance your quality of life and potentially remedy any ailments that you may be suffering from. However, these key benefits can only be achieved if you have an open mind and are willing to try some of the Naturopathy treatments that are available today. Given that many of us are simply used to the traditional medicine that is prevalent in this day and age, Naturopathy principles and philosophies may seem like a new and strange concept. However, you must keep in mind that many of the techniques involved in Naturopathic medicine have been practiced for hundreds, if not thousands, of years throughout the world.

It's a good idea to do your research and find the treatments and practitioners that are right for you and your medical needs. Don't rush into choosing the ideal Naturopath, and ask as many questions as you like. An experienced and trained Naturopath will be more than happy to address any concerns that you may have, and will ensure that you are comfortable with your treatment plan.

Also, be sure to verify that your practitioner is fully licensed and has received an extensive education in the field.

Naturopathy has the power to offer you improved well-being, thanks to the fact that it relies upon your body's own ability to heal itself, and it doesn't include potentially harmful medications or invasive procedures. With Naturopathy, you can use the elements and your body's own energy to remedy health concerns, prevent future medical issues, and enhance your emotional state. With so many benefits, it's not surprising that so many people are now turning to Naturopathy to help them lead a long and happy life.

www.ingramcontent.com/pod-product-compliance
Lightning Source LLC
Chambersburg PA
CBHW050023130526
44590CB00042B/1857